Radiology of Trauma

Radiology of Trauma

Salvatore J.A. Sclafani, MD
Professor of Radiology
State University of New York
Health Sciences Center at Brooklyn
Head, Section of Trauma Radiology
King's County Hospital
Brooklyn, New York

J. B. Lippincott Company • Philadelphia
Gower Medical Publishing • New York • London

Distributed in USA and Canada by:
J.B. Lippincott Company
East Washington Square
Philadelphia, PA 19105
USA

Distributed in the rest of the world (except Japan) by:
Gower Medical Publishing
Middlesex House
34-42 Cleveland Street
London W1P 5FB
UK

Distributed in Japan by:
Nankodo Company Ltd.
42-6, Hongo 3-Chome
Bunkyo-Ku
Tokyo 113
Japan

10 9 8 7 6 5 4 3 2 1

Library of Congress Cataloging-in-Publication Data
Sclafani, Salvatore J. A.
    Radiology of trauma / Salvatore J. A. Sclafani
            p.   cm.
    Includes bibliographical references and index.
    ISBN 1–56375–007–4
    1. Wounds and injuries—Radiography.   2. Diagnostic
imaging.   I. Title.
    [DNLM: 1. Wounds and Injuries—radiography.
2. Diagnostic imaging.   WO 700 S419r]
RD93.7.S35   1991
617.1'40757—dc20
DNLM/DLC
for Library of Congress   91-9622
                                                                      CIP

British Library Cataloguing in Publication Data
Sclafani, Salvatore J. A.
    Radiology of trauma.
    1. Humans. Injuries. Radiology.
    I. Title
    617.10757
    ISBN 1–56375–007–4

Editors: Bill Gabello, Patrick D. O'Neill
Art Director: Jill Feltham
Illustrator: Alan Landau, Seward Hung
Designer: Nava Anav
Layout: Lori Thorn

Printed in Hong Kong
Produced by Mandarin Offset

CONTENTS

SECTION I:

Radiology of Skeletal Trauma

Radiologic Examination of the Trauma Patient

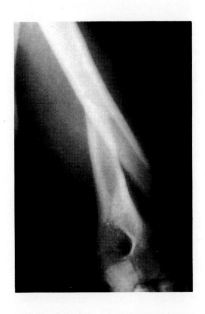

The primary aim of radiologic examination of the trauma patient is to identify life threatening but clinically occult injuries. Certain fractures, such as fractures of the pelvis and the cervical spine, fall into this category. When such fractures are suspected, radiographic studies are done early, often with portable equipment. Most fractures, however, are not life threatening, and radiologic evaluation can generally be deferred until more pressing injuries have been assessed and the patient has been stabilized.

Secondary aims of radiographic examination are to provide additional anatomic and pathologic information about clinically evident injuries and to generate baseline images before definitive therapy is begun. Although examinations done for either of these purposes are often valuable, or even essential, they should not be allowed to delay treatment of more important injuries, nor should they subject the patient to unnecessary risk or pain, or entail movement of the fracture site. The injured area should be splinted during transit; however, the splint should be removed before the films are taken, since it is likely to obscure the area of interest, especially if it is made of plaster.

A single projection of a suspected fracture site is seldom sufficient: a fracture or dislocation can be missed, and even if it is detected, the extent and character of the injury may be unclear. Certain injuries are commonly accompanied by an additional fracture or dislocation that may be some distance from the clinically evident fracture. It is therefore necessary to visualize the joints both proximal and distal to the fracture. For example, to evaluate an ankle fracture properly, the radiologist must obtain radiographs of the entire leg, including the knee joint.

INDICATORS OF FRACTURE

The presence of a fracture is indicated by a break in or abrupt angulation of the cortex, discontinuity of the bony trabeculae, a radiolucent fracture line, or increased density due to overlapping fragments. Deep soft-tissue swelling or distortion of landmarks (e.g., displacement of the extraarticular elbow fat pad or obliteration of normal fascical stripes) should arouse suspicion even when the bone appears intact. Joint swelling due to intraarticular blood is often seen in fractures that involve the intraarticular portion of a bone. An intraarticular fat–fluid level is unequivocal evidence of a fracture, but it is only demonstrable on a horizontal-beam (i.e., "cross-table") projection (Fig. 1.1).

Radiologic analysis of a fracture does not end with detection of the injury: one must also define the characteristics of the fracture. Many different terms are used for classifying fractures. A fracture may, for instance, be incomplete, meaning that it does not completely disrupt the continuity of the bone; isolated, meaning that it is not associated with any other fractures; comminuted (Fig. 1.2), meaning that the bone is splintered or crushed; or segmental (Fig. 1.3), meaning that the bone is fractured in two places. A fracture may be open (compound) or closed, depending on whether it produces an open wound in the skin or not. Evaluated on the basis of the direction of the break, a fracture may be transverse (Fig. 1.4), meaning that the break extends at right angles to the axis of the bone; oblique (Fig. 1.5), meaning that the break extends in an oblique direction; spiral (Fig. 1.6), meaning that the bone has been twisted apart; or impacted, meaning that one fragment has been driven into the other. Depending on where in the bone the break occurs, a fracture may be epiphyseal, metaphyseal, diaphyseal, intraarticular, or nonarticular. The Salter-Harris classification (Fig. 1.7) is useful for fractures involving the growth plate (physis) in children and adolescents. A fracture may also be associated with a joint dislocation or subluxation (Fig. 1.8).

Furthermore, the fragments (segments) created by a fracture may be displaced or angulated (Fig. 1.9). They may overlap, causing shortening of the bone (Fig. 1.10), or they may be widely separated (distracted). Finally, fractures can be classified according to the circumstances of their genesis, whether through preexisting lesions (pathologic fractures; Fig. 1.11); in bone weakened by a generalized disorder, such as osteoporosis (insufficiency fractures); or in bone subjected to excessive stress (stress fractures).

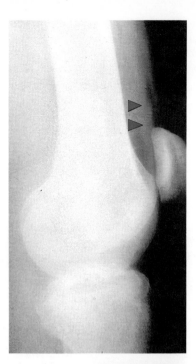

Fig. 1.1 Lipohemarthrosis. *A cross-table lateral film of the knee shows a fat/fluid level* (arrows) *in the knee joint. Intraarticular marrow and blood will layer because fat is less dense than blood. Although the fracture site is not visible on the film, this sign is a reliable indicator of an intraarticular fracture. One should look carefully for subtle signs of fracture on other projections. Special studies such as tomography or bone scan may be needed to demonstrate the fracture.*

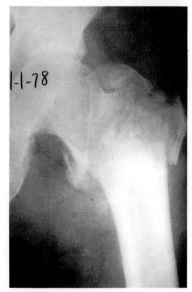

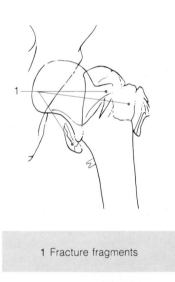

1 Fracture fragments

Fig. 1.2 Comminuted fracture. *Frontal projection of the hip shows a comminuted fracture of the intertrochanteric region of the femur; that is, there are multiple fracture fragments.*

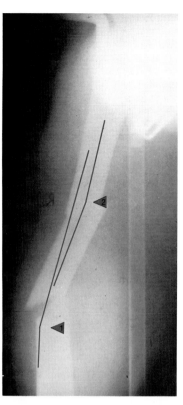

Fig. 1.3 Segmental fracture. *Frontal projection of the leg shows two fractures of the tibia. This injury is classified as a segmental fracture because each fracture extends through both cortices. Angulation is determined by the angle between the proximal* (uppermost) *and the distal* (lower-most) *fragment* (arrow 1), *not by the angle between the proximal and the central fragment* (arrow 2). *Thus, whereas there is lateral angulation of the central fragment with respect to the proximal fragment, and medial angulation of the distal fragment with respect to the central fragment, this should be described as "medial angulation of the distal fragment with respect to the proximal fragment."*

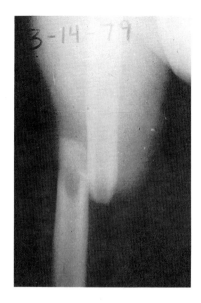

Fig. 1.5 Oblique shaft fracture. *Frontal projection of the thigh shows an oblique fracture of the femoral shaft. There is no angulation, but the distal fragment is laterally displaced.*

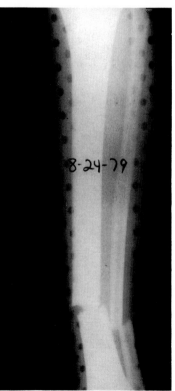

Fig. 1.4 Transverse shaft fractures. *Frontal projection of the leg in a splint shows transverse fractures of the distal shaft of the tibia and fibula. Both fractures are slightly angulated. When describing angulation, one must give a reference point: For example, this fracture can be described as either "lateral angulation of the distal fragment" or "medial angulation of the fracture apex." Simply describing it as "medial" or "lateral" angulation is inadequate.*

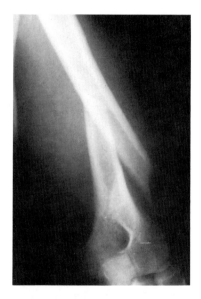

Fig. 1.6 Spiral oblique fracture. *Frontal projection of the arm shows a spiral oblique fracture of the humeral shaft. The distal fragment is displaced medially and angulated medially.*

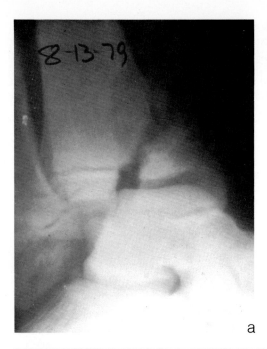

Fig. 1.7 Salter–Harris IV fracture. *a* *Oblique projection of the ankle in a teenager shows a fracture of the tibia traversing the epiphysis, physis (growth plate), and metaphysis. The fracture extends into the joint, causing incongruity of the articular surface.* ***b*** *The Salter–Harris classification is very useful for analyzing growth-plate fractures. The rare Type V injury is a crush injury of the physis that is usually caused by a fall from a height.*

a

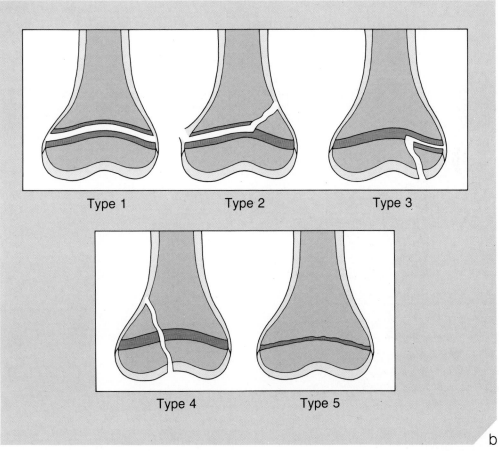

Type 1   Type 2   Type 3

Type 4   Type 5

b

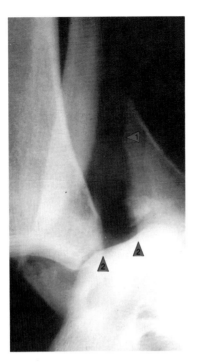

Fig. 1.8 Fracture-dislocation of the ankle. *Lateral projection of the ankle shows a displaced oblique fracture of the distal fibula* (arrow 1) *and a posterior dislocation of the talus. The articular surface of the talus is indicated* (arrows 2).

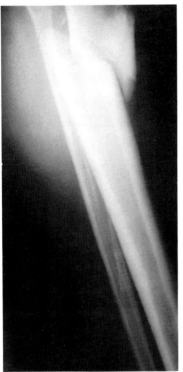

Fig. 1.9 Oblique fracture with recurvatum deformity. *Lateral projection of the leg shows an oblique fracture with posterior displacement and anterior angulation of the distal fragment. This anterior angulation is also called* recurvatum *because it reverses the normal curvature of the tibia. The obliquity of the fracture line suggests instability.*

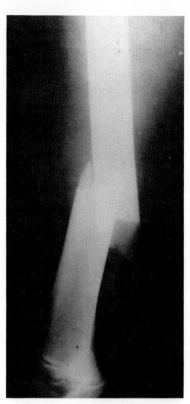

Fig. 1.10 Transverse fracture with shortening. *Lateral projection of the thigh shows a transverse fracture of the midfemur. There is shortening due to overlapping of the fracture fragments, and anterior angulation of the distal fragment.*

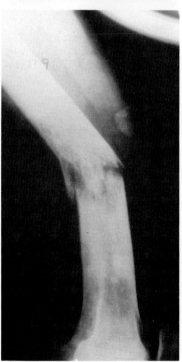

Fig. 1.11 Pathologic fracture secondary to metastatic carcinoma. *Lateral projection of the thigh shows a transverse fracture of the femoral shaft with posterior angulation of the distal fragment. The fracture has occurred through an area of motheaten destruction typical of bone metastasis. The patient had carcinoma of the breast with widespread bone metastases.*

CHAPTER TWO

*F*ractures of the Face and Skull

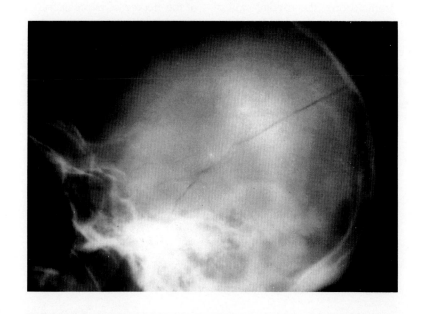

FACIAL FRACTURES

Facial injuries are not usually life-threatening and are often given secondary priority in the radiographic evaluation of a patient with multiple injuries. Nonetheless, a limited radiographic survey should be performed initially in such cases, followed by a more thorough examination when the patient is more stable. Complete radiologic evaluation of facial trauma requires multiple projections (Fig. 2.1), supplemented by pluridirectional (thin-section) tomography or computed tomography (CT) in selected cases. Since tomography and CT expose the radiosensitive lens to additional radiation, they should be omitted unless it is clear that the additional information they provide will significantly affect management decisions. Of the two, CT is preferred, since it not only delineates both soft tissues and bony structures but also subjects the lens to less radiation than pluridirectional tomography does.

Fractures of the nasal bones may be simple and nondisplaced, depressed, comminuted, or complex. They may be associated with fractures of the maxilla, the frontal bone, the medial wall of the orbit, or the nasal septum. Nasal fractures are best seen on lateral nasal views (Figs. 2.2, 2.3) and on the Waters projection.

Blowout fractures of the orbital floor are caused by increased intraorbital pressure, such as may result from the impact of a ball, fist, or other hard object on the globe. As the globe is displaced into the orbit, the weakest portion of the orbit (usually the orbital floor) breaks. The most common radiographic finding is clouding of the maxillary antrum. When the fracture is visible, it may appear as multiple small or linear fragments (which are often displaced into the maxillary antrum). The anterior portion of the orbital floor is best seen on the Waters projection, where as the posterior portion is best seen on the Caldwell projection (Fig. 2.4). In the Caldwell projection, the posterior aspect of the floor resembles a chaise longue, with the back of the "chair" in an erect position. When a fracture occurs in that region, the "back of the chair" is in the recumbent position. Sometimes it is impossible to visualize the fracture itself, because the floor has been comminuted into tiny fragments that are obscured by the surrounding soft-tissue swelling (Fig. 2.5). Pluridirectional tomography and CT are useful if management of the patient requires precise localization of the fracture and measurement of the degree of depression. CT is indicated if the status of the globe or extraocular muscles is in doubt (Fig. 2.6).

Fractures of the malar complex, also called tripod fractures, are usually caused by a direct blow to the cheek. The classic tripod fracture involves the palpable orbital rim, the lateral orbital wall (usually the frontozygomatic suture or the frontal process of the zygoma), and the lateral wall of the maxillary antrum. Associated fractures involve the orbital floor and the zygomatic arch. The malar eminence is displaced posteriorly, inferiorly, and medially (Figs. 2.7, 2.8).

Zygomatic arch fractures may be occult; consequently, demonstration of their presence often requires meticulous radiographic technique. These fractures are best seen on a slightly oblique submentovertex projection, which allows clear visualization of the comminution and depression of the fragments (Fig. 2.9a,b). (A view of the uninjured side should be obtained for comparison.) On the Waters projection the zygomatic arch projects from the malar bone in such a way that it resembles an elephant trunk; when the arch is disrupted, the "elephant's trunk" is not seen (Fig. 2.9c). An associated mandibular fracture, usually of the coronoid process, is not uncommon.

A fracture of the superior orbital rim may result from injury to the forehead of the sort caused by a blow from a heavy object or by direct impact with a windshield of an automobile.

The fracture is best seen in the Caldwell projection, though oblique views may be helpful in some instances (Fig. 2.10). When these fractures extend into the frontal sinus, it is important to determine if they extend through the posterior wall as an open skull fracture. Axial CT is the best method for determining this.

LeFort fractures are complex fractures in which segments of the face are separated from the skull. The loss of these supports renders the face unstable, and operative repair is essential to restore normal function and appearance. There is often an associated cranial fracture or intracranial injury; a cerebrospinal fluid leak or carotid-cavernous fistula may develop in some patients. LeFort described three areas of intrinsic weakness that are prone to fracture. Each area corresponds to a specific type of LeFort fracture. LeFort I fracture lines extend transversely through the maxilla, separating the hard palate from the remaining face and skull; LeFort II fractures pass through the midface, separating the nasomaxillary complex from the rest of the face; and LeFort III fracture lines separate the entire face from the skull (Fig. 2.11). In reality, "pure" I, II, or III fractures are rare: most patients present with a combination of two or more fracture patterns. Although LeFort fractures are easily diagnosed on plain films (Fig. 2.12), more sophisticated studies (tomography or CT) are needed to characterize the fracture pattern and plan reconstruction.

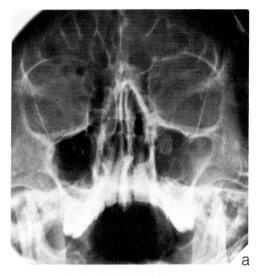

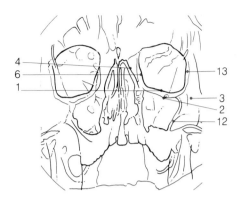

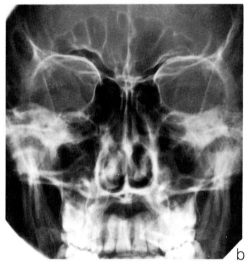

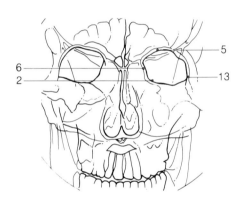

Fig. 2.1 Multiple projections of facial trauma. *a Normal Waters projection. b Normal Caldwell projection. c Normal Townes projection. d Normal submentovertex (base) projection. e Normal lateral projection of mandible.*

1 Orbital rim	9 Angle of mandible
2 Orbital floor	10 Horizontal mandibular ramus
3 Zygoma	
4 Nasal bone	11 Coronoid process
5 Supraorbital rim	12 Lateral maxillary wall
6 Medial orbital wall	
7 Mandibular condyle	13 Lateral orbital wall
8 Ascending mandibular ramus	

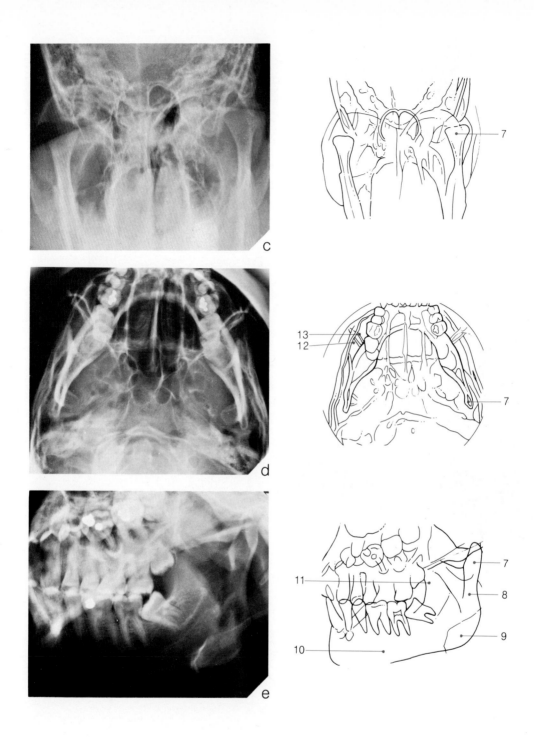

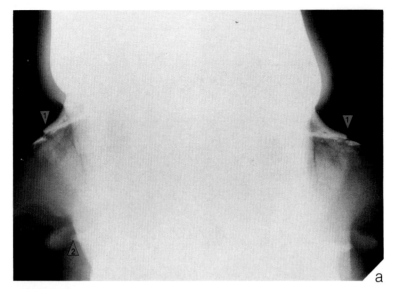

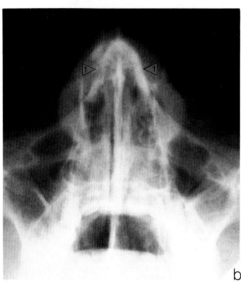

Fig. 2.2 Isolated nasal fracture. *a Lateral and* **b** *Waters projection show a fracture (arrows 1) of the nasal bones at the bridge of the nose with marked depression of the fragments. The anterior nasal spine (arrow 2) of the maxilla is not fractured.*

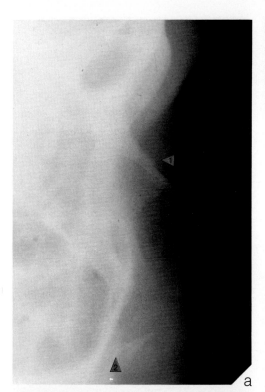

Fig. 2.3 Nasal fracture associated with complex facial fractures. *a* Lateral projection shows a comminuted fracture (arrow 1) of the nasal bone, which is not depressed. The anterior nasal spine is fractured (arrow 2). ***b*** Waters view shows medial displacement of the nasal bone (arrow). Other views showed fractures of the maxillary alveolus, posterior orbital floor, and zygoma.

a

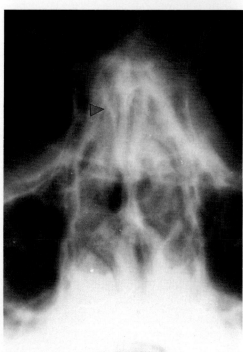

b

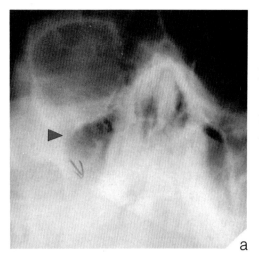

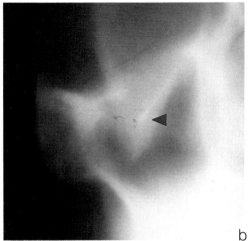

Fig. 2.4 Fracture of floor of orbit. *a Waters view reveals opacification of the right maxillary antrum* (arrow), *but a fracture cannot be identified. b Frontal thin-section tomogram clearly demonstrates a "trap door" fracture that is hinged medially* (arrow). *The fragment is markedly depressed. c In a patient with a left orbital floor fracture, the Caldwell view shows that the "chaise longue" is in the recumbent position* (arrows) *indicating that the posterior part of the floor is fractured.*

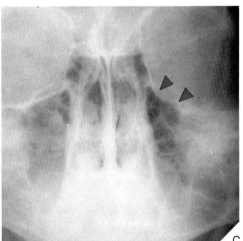

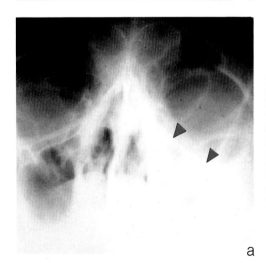

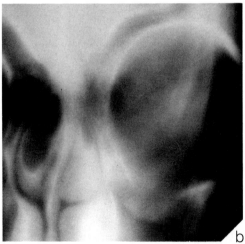

Fig. 2.5 Blowout fracture of orbital floor. *a Waters view shows opacification of the left maxillary antrum. The fracture cannot be iden-* tified. *The orbital rim* (arrows) *is intact. b A thin-section tomogram clearly shows the extensive blowout fracture of the orbital floor.*

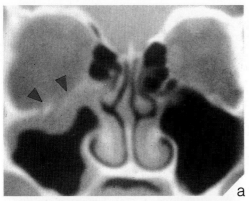

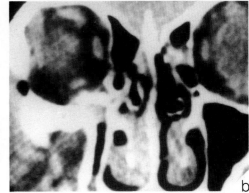

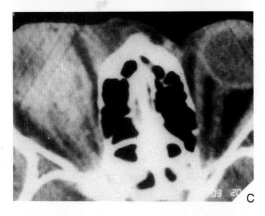

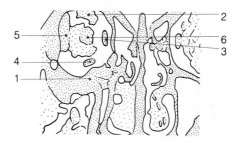

Fig. 2.6 Blowout fracture of orbital floor.
a Coronal CT scan shows a large orbital floor fracture (arrows) with downward herniation of orbital soft tissues. *b* Soft-tissue display shows no evidence of herniation or entrapment of extraocular muscles. *c* In another patient with a blowout fracture an axial CT cut shows a retrobulbar, intraconal hematoma in the right orbit (compare with normal left orbit). An intraconal hematoma results in increased intraconal pressure, which may cause retinal artery occlusion, and represents an acute surgical emergency.

1 Orbital floor fracture	4 Inferior rectus muscle
2 Superior rectus muscle	5 Lateral rectus muscle
3 Medial rectus muscle	6 Optic nerve

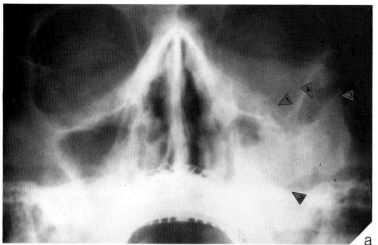

Fig. 2.7 Tripod fracture of the maxilla. *a* Waters view shows inferior displacement of the malar bone. There are fractures of the palpable inferior orbital rim (arrow 1) *and the* lateral wall of the maxilla (arrow 2), together with disruption of the fronto-zygomatic (arrow 3) and spheno-zygomatic (arrow 4) sutures. There is also a fracture of the orbital floor. *b* Waters view of another patient shows inferior displacement of the malar eminence and angulation of the lateral wall of the maxillary sinus. *c* Submentovertex (base) projection in a third patient shows posterior displacement (arrows) of left malar complex.

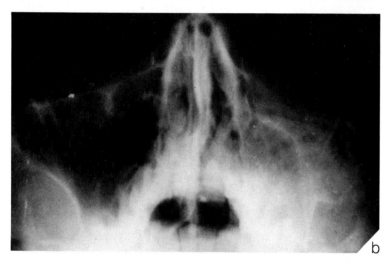

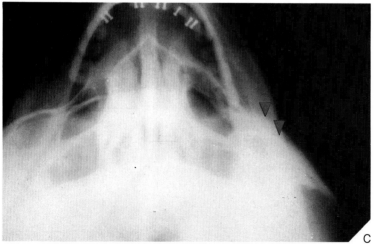

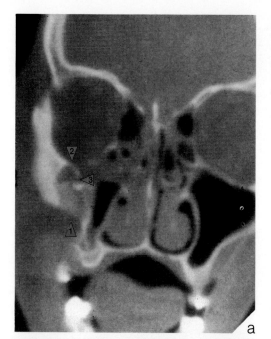

a

Fig. 2.8 Tripod fracture of the maxilla.
a Coronal CT scan shows fractures of the lateral maxillary wall (arrow 1), the orbital rim (arrow 2), and the orbital floor (arrow 3). *b* Axial slice shows fractures of the anterior maxillary wall, posterolateral maxillary wall, and the body of the zygoma. The right maxillary sinus is opaque (filled with blood), and there is an air-fluid level in the left maxillary sinus.

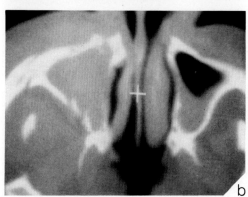

b

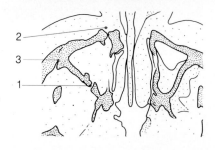

1 Fracture of lateral maxillary wall	3 Fracture of zygoma
2 Fracture of anterior wall of maxillary sinus	

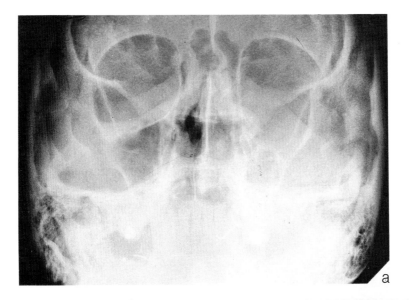

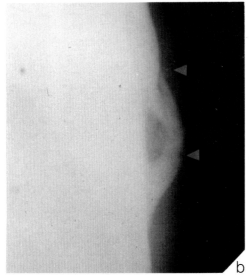

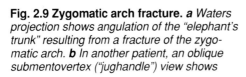

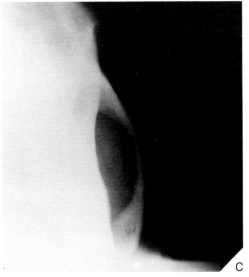

Fig. 2.9 Zygomatic arch fracture. *a* Waters projection shows angulation of the "elephant's trunk" resulting from a fracture of the zygomatic arch. *b* In another patient, an oblique submentovertex ("jughandle") view shows a fracture of the zygoma (arrows) with marked depression of the left zygomatic arch. *c* Compare the preceding with the smooth, continuous appearance of the normal right zygomatic arch.

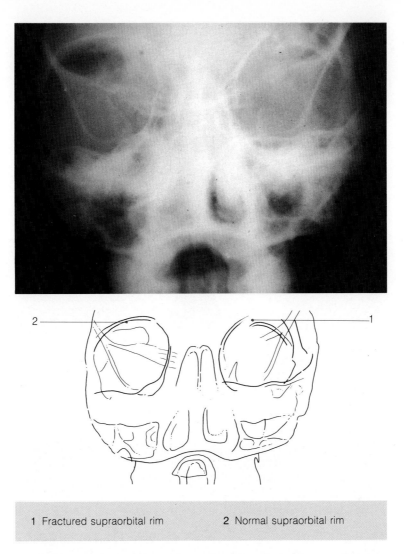

| 1 Fractured supraorbital rim | 2 Normal supraorbital rim |

Fig. 2.10 Fracture of superior orbital rim. *Caldwell projection shows an angulated superior orbital rim fracture on the left. Compare normal orbital contour on the right.*

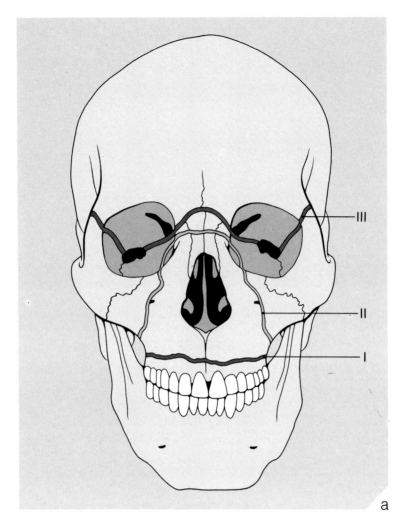

a

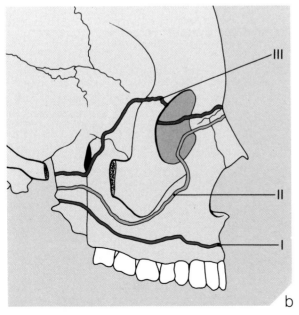

b

Fig. 2.11 LeFort fractures of the face.
a, b LeFort I fractures separate the maxillary alve-olus from the remainder of the face. LeFort II frac-tures are located in the middle of the face and separate the nasomaxillary complex from the remainder of the face. LeFort III fractures separate the entire face from the skull. "Pure" LeFort frac-tures are not common; most patients have a com-bination of the three types. Both tomography and CT may be needed for comprehensive analysis.

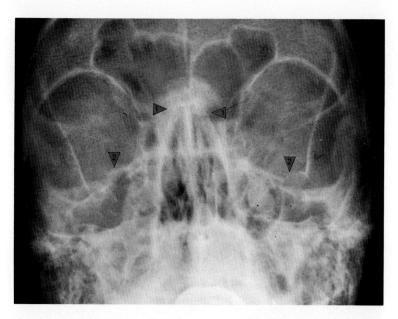

Fig. 2.12 LeFort fracture. *Waters projection shows that the face is separated from the skull in the midline at the nasofrontal junction* (arrows 1) *and laterally through both frontozygomatic sutures. There are also displaced fractures of the palpable rims of both orbits. LeFort fractures almost always involve the floor of the orbit as well* (arrows 2).

MANDIBULAR FRACTURES

The mandible is composed of two mirror-image structures that unite anteriorly at the midline. Each half has a horizontal ramus, or body, and a vertical ramus. The vertical ramus has two processes: the coronoid and the condyle. The condyle articulates with the glenoid fossa of the temporal bone. The mandible forms a ring; consequently, as with all ring structures, fractures usually occur in at least two places. Discovery of an isolated mandibular fracture should therefore be viewed with skepticism. Appropriate radiologic studies are necessary to determine whether there is an additional fracture or dislocation. Associated injuries of the cervical spine and face are not uncommon and must be ruled out.

In evaluating mandibular trauma, one must consider the following important factors: the location of the fracture, the angle of the fracture lines, the presence or absence of teeth on each side of the fracture, potential involvement of teeth or roots in the fracture, and the presence of preexisting dental pathology (Figs. 2.13–2.17).

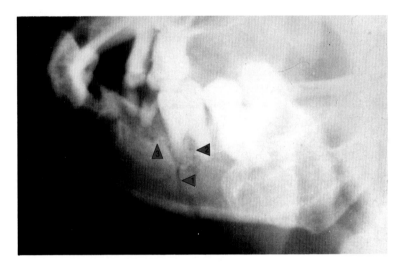

Fig. 2.13 Class I horizontal ramus fracture. *Oblique projection of the mandible shows an undisplaced vertical fracture* (arrow 1) *through the horizontal ramus of the mandible. The presence of teeth in the posterior fragment inhibits superior displacement. Note that the fracture extends into the root* (arrow 2) *and is adjacent to a periapical abscess* (arrow 3).

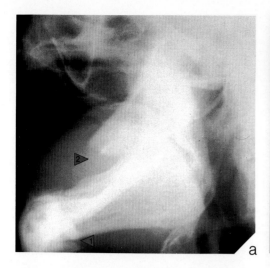

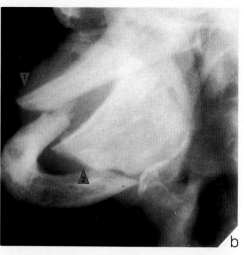

Fig. 2.14 Class III fractures of the edentulous mandible. *a Lateral and b oblique projections show fractures of the symphysis (arrows 1) and the horizontal rami (arrows 2). The symphysis and the horizontal rami are displaced inferiorly and posteriorly. There are no teeth to use as posts for stabilization of the fracture fragments.*

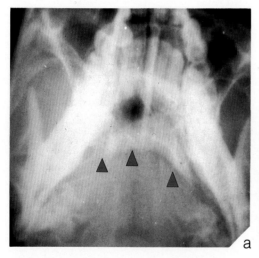

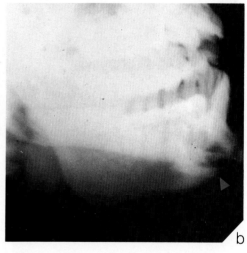

Fig. 2.15 Parasymphyseal fractures.
a Frontal and b oblique projections of the mandible show comminuted parasymphyseal fractures (arrows). The muscles of the tongue attach to this area of the mandible, when a fracture is present, the tongue may be displaced posteriorly, which can result in airway obstruction.

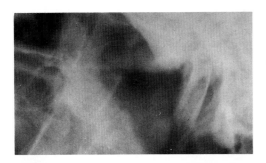

Fig. 2.16 Fracture of mandibular condyle.
Lateral projection shows a fracture of the base of the mandibular condyle with anterior displacement of the ramus.

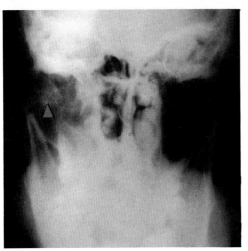

Fig. 2.17 Fracture of mandibular condyle.
Posteroanterior projection of the face shows that the right mandibular condyle is fractured and dislocated lingually (arrow). This finding is best seen on the Townes projection.

SKULL FRACTURES

Skull radiographs are often—probably excessively—used to identify skull fractures (Fig. 2.18). Because the presence (or absence) of a fracture does not predict the presence (or absence) of an intracranial injury, CT is the preferred modality for initial examination of a patient with head trauma. (If skull films are obtained, the relation of the fracture to the vascular grooves should be carefully observed, since fractures that cross vascular grooves may be associated with epidural hemorrhage.) Skull radiographs are still of great value in patients with scalp lacerations, penetrating wounds, or possible depressed fracture (Fig. 2.19a). In patients with depressed fractures, CT should be performed to determine the degree of depression and to rule out underlying intracranial pathology (Fig. 2.19b).

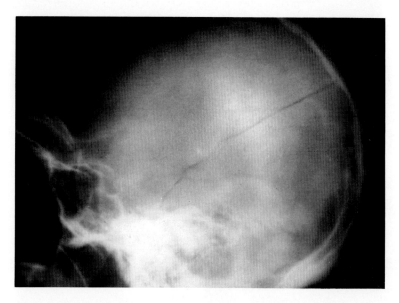

Fig. 2.18 Linear skull fracture. *Lateral projection shows a sharp, jagged, nonbranching linear radiolucency in the parietal bone.*

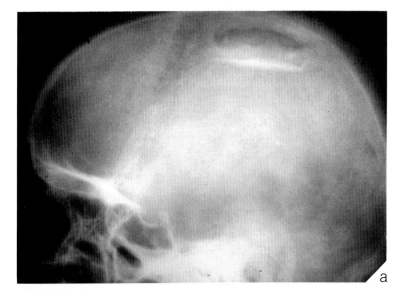

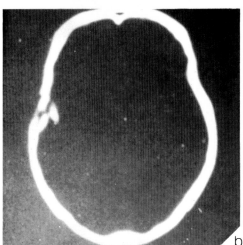

Fig. 2.19 Depressed skull fracture. *a* A depressed fracture of the parietal bone is seen as a double density adjacent to a lucency on a lateral skull film. *b* Axial CT (bone display) shows the depressed fragments.

CHAPTER THREE

Fractures of the
Spinal Column

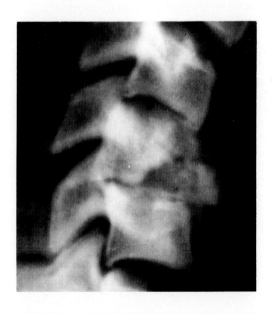

EXAMINATION OF THE CERVICAL SPINE

The cervical spine should be the first area studied in a patient who has sustained multiple injuries, because cervical spine stability must be established before the neck can be moved or the patient transferred to another area. If it is necessary to move or transport an unstable patient before radiologic clearance is granted, the patient's neck must be securely immobilized.

After major trauma, the initial radiographic study should be performed with portable equipment. The first film obtained should be a supine cross-table lateral view with the shoulders depressed. Depression of the shoulders is essential to ensure that the lower cervical spine is not obscured by the dense shoulder muscles; it is accomplished by pulling the arms downward while an assistant holds the patient's head stationary (Fig. 3.1). If all seven vertebrae are not visualized, a second attempt should be made with additional traction.

If C7 is still not adequately visualized (and this is not uncommon), it is preferable to attempt different views rather than repeat the cross-table lateral projection a third time. The "swimmer's lateral" projection (with one arm extended above the head), conventional tomography, and computed tomography have all been recommended, but in my experience a series of plain films in the frontal and oblique projections is usually sufficient to exclude unstable fractures and dislocations and subluxations. Two frontal views are obtained: one with the x-ray beam (central ray) angled toward the head, the second with the x-ray beam angled toward the feet (Fig. 3.2). This pair of frontal projections allows the radiologist to assess the status of the vertebral bodies and the posterior elements. Two cross-table oblique views, which allow further inspection of the pedicles and facets, complete the examination (Fig. 3.3). Additional studies, such as lateral flexion/extension films, right and left bending frontal films, conventional tomography, computed tomography, and myelography may be indicated in selected cases.

Evaluation of alignment in the lateral projection requires analysis of three imaginary lines: The first line runs along the anterior aspect of the vertebral bodies; the second line runs along the posterior aspect of the vertebral bodies; and the third line runs along the posterior aspect of the spinal canal at the junctions of the laminae and the spinous processes (the spinolaminal line) (Fig. 3.4). These imaginary lines should slope gently from one vertebra to the next; the distance between two adjoining spinous processes should also be consistent throughout.

Prevertebral soft-tissue swelling due to hemorrhage is a common finding in cervical spine injuries. In adults and older children, the thickness of the soft tissues between the anterior aspect of C4 and the posterior aspect of the hypopharyngeal airway should be no greater than 40 percent of the anteroposterior diameter of the body of C4. The vertebral bodies should be equal in height from C3 through C7, and the cortical margins of each vertebral bone should be sharp and well-defined. At each level, the inferior facets of a given vertebra should be posterior to the superior facets of the vertebra just below it. In frontal views, the lateral edges of the vertebra should align with one another. The vertebral end-plates should be seen as a sharp line, and the intervertebral disc spaces should not differ significantly in height from one to the next. The oblique views, though difficult to interpret, provide useful information about the pedicles, facets, and lamina. If the odontoid process of C2 is not well visualized on these films, "open mouth" frontal views can be taken; these usually demonstrate this area adequately.

It is essential to remember that a single complete view of the cervical spine does not constitute an adequate radiographic examination: Visualization of the entire cervical spine must be achieved in at least two projections (Fig. 3.5).

The common injuries to which the cervical spine is subject include the following:

1. Atlantoaxial subluxation, which involves an increase in the space between Cl and C2 (Fig. 3.6);
2. Fractures of the odontoid (Fig. 3.7);
3. Fractures of the pedicles of C2 (Fig. 3.8);
4. Fractures of the transverse process (Fig. 3.9), which are increasingly common in automotive collisions when shoulder harness seatbelts are worn;
5. Hyperextension injury, which is often associated with various types of fractures (Figs. 3.10, 3.11);
6. Hyperflexion injury, which is also often associated with fractures (Fig. 3.12); but in some cases is associated with subluxation without fracture (Fig. 3.13);
7. Dislocations of the facets of the vertebrae (Fig. 3.14).

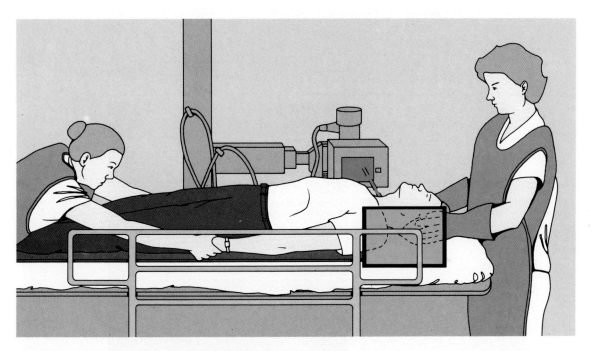

Fig. 3.1 Cross-table lateral projection of the cervical spine. *While an assistant stabilizes the patient's head, downward traction is applied to depress the shoulders, the muscles of which may obscure the lower cervical spine. The film is obtained with a horizontal x-ray beam.*

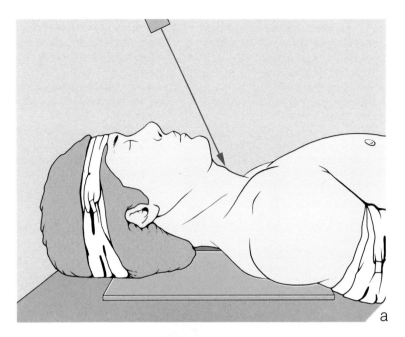

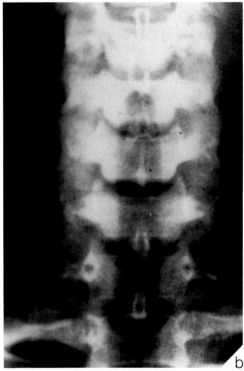

Fig. 3.2 Anteroposterior projections of the cervical spine. *Examination of the cervical spine begins with two frontal views, one an anteroposterior view with cephalic angulation (a,b), the other an anteroposterior view with caudal angulation (c,d).*

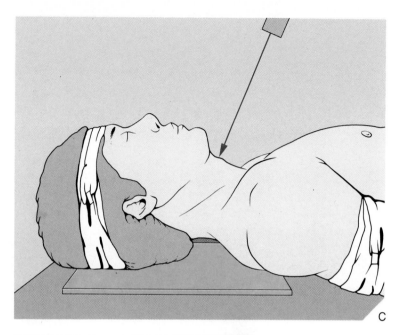

c

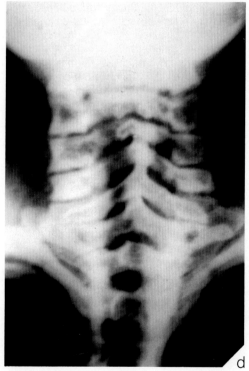

d

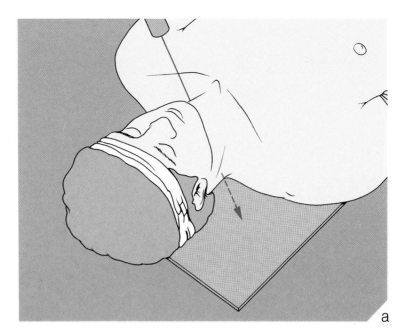

Fig. 3.3 Supine oblique projection of the
cervical spine. *After frontal views are
obtained, examination of the cervical spine
continues with cross-table oblique views (**a,b**).*

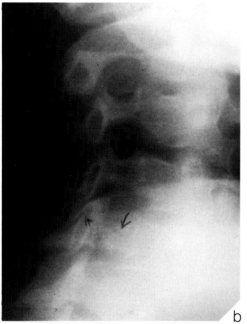

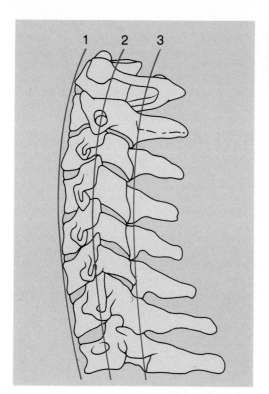

Fig. 3.4 Contour lines of the cervical spine.
Line 1 *follows the anterior aspect of the verte-bral bodies,* line 2 *the posterior aspect of the vertebral bodies, and* line 3 *the junctions between the laminae and the spinous process-es on the posterior aspect of the spinal canal.*

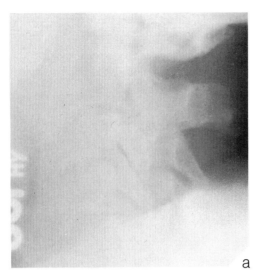

a

Fig. 3.5 Missed fracture due to inadequate radiographic examination. *An adequate radiographic examination must allow visualization of the entire cervical spine in at least two projections.* **a** *This lateral radiograph of an injured motorcyclist was interpreted as "a limited but grossly normal examination." This interpretation is incorrect. The lateral film shown here is unsatisfactory and therefore nondiagnostic: no conclusions can be drawn about the integrity of the vertebra below C4.* **b** *The initial AP film shows discontinuity (arrows) of the end-plates of the body of C6, caused by vertical compression. This finding went unrecognized, and the patient was discharged after treatment of his wrist fracture.* **c** *A repeat examination performed two months later because of progressive quadriparesis shows a hyperflexion fracture of C6 with posterior subluxation of C5.*

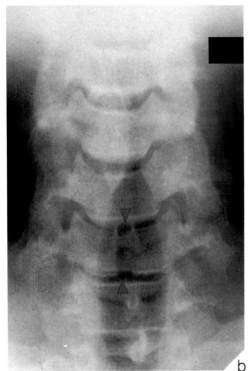

b

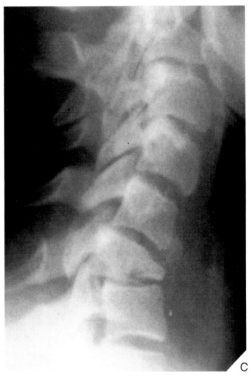

c

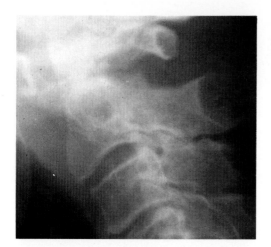

Fig. 3.6 Atlantoaxial subluxation. *Lateral projection of the upper cervical spine shows that the space between the posterior aspect of the anterior arch of Cl and the anterior aspect of the odontoid process measures 4 mm (normal, 2 mm or less). The spinolaminal junction of C1 is displaced anteriorly with respect to the other vertebrae. Traumatic atlantoaxial subluxation results from a tear of the transverse ligament.*

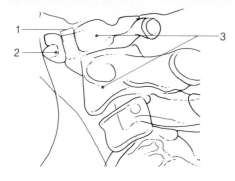

1 Increased distance between C1 and C2	2 Ring of atlas
	3 Odontoid

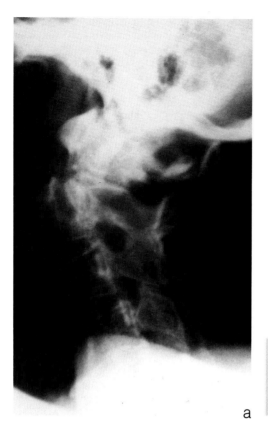

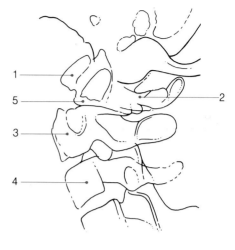

1 Ring of C1	**4** C3
2 Posterior elements of C1	**5** Fracture of odontoid
3 C2	

a

Fig. 3.7 Odontoid fracture. *a Lateral projection shows that the odontoid and C1 are displaced posteriorly to the rest of the cervical spine. b Anteroposterior tomogram shows a fracture through the base of the odontoid (arrows 5).*

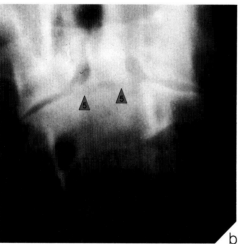

b

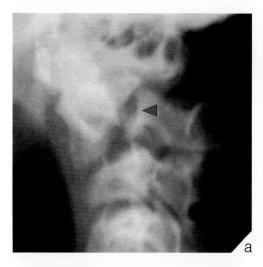

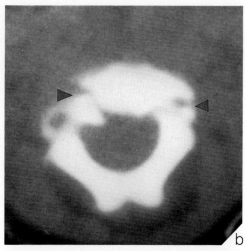

Fig. 3.8 Hangman fracture. *a Lateral projection shows anterior displacement of the body of C2 and a fracture* (arrow) *through the pedicles.*

b In another patient an axial CT scan shows fractures (arrows) *of both pedicles.*

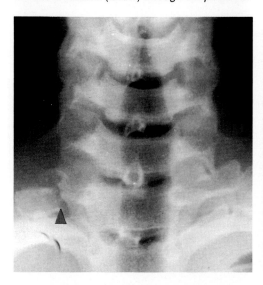

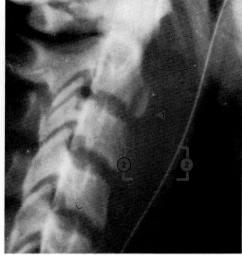

Fig. 3.9 Transverse process fracture. *This man complained of neck pain after his automobile was struck from the rear. An anteroposterior projection of the cervical spine shows an undisplaced fracture* (arrow) *through the right transverse process of C7. Transverse process fractures may be associated with a brachial plexus nerve injury as well as with dislocation or fracture of the first rib.*

Fig. 3.10 Hyperextension teardrop fracture. *Lateral projection shows an avulsion fracture* (arrow 1) *of the attachment of the anterior longitudinal ligament. Note the extensive prevertebral hematoma* (braces 2), *which has widened the space between the spine and the posterior aspect of the airway. This space should not be more than 40 percent of the anteroposterior diameter of the body of C4.*

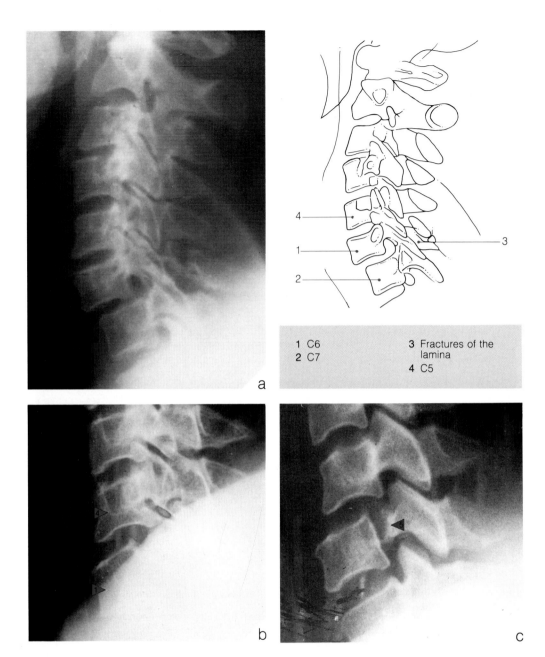

1 C6	3 Fractures of the
2 C7	lamina
	4 C5

Fig. 3.11 Hyperextension injury with fracture of posterior elements. *a* During hyperextension the posterior elements impinge upon each other and may fracture. Fractures may occur through the pedicles, the lamina, or both. In this lateral projection, C6 is anteriorly subluxated on C7 and there are fractures of the laminae of C6 and C7. ***b,c*** This pair of lateral films in another patient with a hyperextension injury illustrates the value of a complete radiographic examination. The initial film (***b***) shows apparent posterior subluxation of C5 (arrow 4). The patient's shoulders obscure the body and posterior elements of C6 (arrow 1). A repeat film with downward traction on the arms (***c***) shows a fracture (arrow 5) through the base of the pedicles of C6 that has rendered the spine unstable.

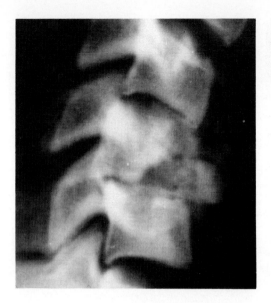

Fig. 3.12 Hyperflexion fracture. *Lateral film shows loss of the normal cervical lordosis. The C5 vertebral body is crushed, split and impacted. The facet joints and the interspinous distance are widened at the same level.*

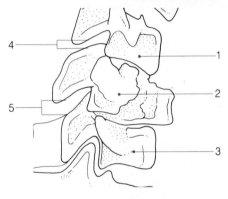

1 C4	4 C4–C5 interspinous distance
2 C5	
3 C6	5 C5–C6 interspinous distance

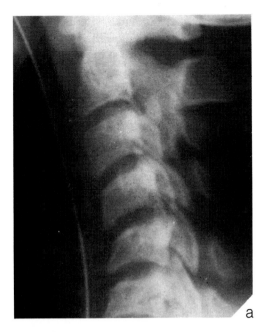

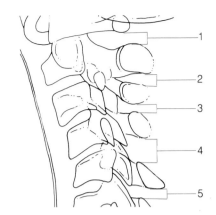

1 C1–C2 interspinous distance	4 C4–C5 interspinous distance
2 C2–C3 interspinous distance	5 C5–C6 interspinous distance
3 C3–C4 distance	

Fig. 3.13 Hyperflexion injury showing subluxation without fracture. *a Lateral projection of a patient with a hyperflexion injury shows no fracture, but there is loss of the normal cervical lordosis. The distances between adjacent spinous processes (interspinous distances) are identical at all levels except at C4–C5. Widening of the interspinous distance at C4–C5 indicates disruption of ligamentous support at this level, with resultant instability. b,c In another patient with a hyperflexion injury, the initial lateral projection (b) shows* normal alignment. Because the patient complained of considerable neck pain, a repeat film was obtained with active flexion (*c*). The repeat film shows widening of the interspinous distance between C4 and C5 (braces 4), indicating ligamentous instability. Flexion and extension views should always be done actively; that is, the patient should move his or her own neck to tolerance (provided that no neurologic signs or symptoms develop). One should never try to obtain flexion and extension views by passively manipulating the patient's neck.

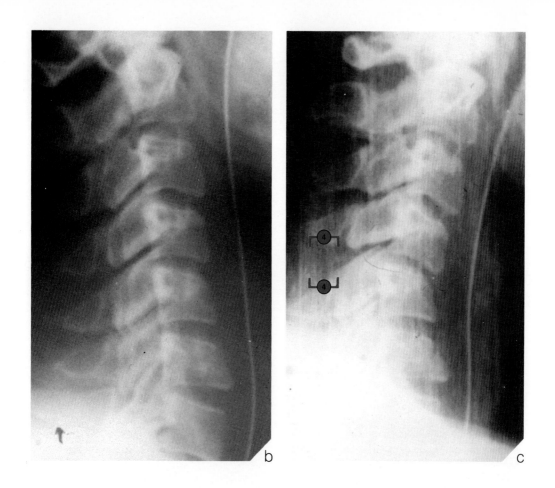

b

c

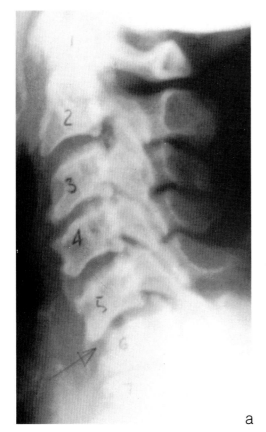
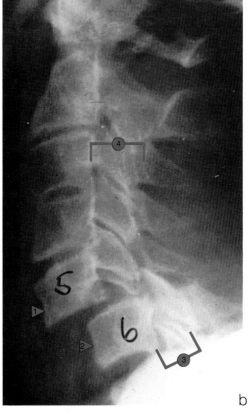

a

b

Fig. 3.14 Facet dislocations. *a* Lateral projection shows a unilateral "jumped" facet. C5 is markedly subluxated anteriorly, and the C5–C6 interspinous space is widened. One of the inferior facets of C5 is perched on the superior facet of C6. Note that C1–C5 appear to be in a steep oblique projection, whereas C6 appears to be in a true lateral projection. *b* Lateral film of another patient shows bilateral locked facets, with C5 (arrow 1) dislocated anteriorly to C6 (arrow 2). Both inferior facets of C5 are displaced anterior to the superior facets of C6. The vertebral canal (brace 3) between the posterior aspect of the C6 vertebral body and the spinolaminal junction is markedly narrowed, resulting in compression of the spinal cord. Compare normal width of spinal canal at C3 (brace 4).

EXAMINATION OF THE THORACIC AND LUMBOSACRAL SPINE

For evaluation of the thoracic spine, frontal and lateral projections are usually sufficient, and additional films are rarely needed. For assessment of the lumbosacral spine, frontal and lateral views are generally sufficient; however an additional lateral film with the x-ray beam centered at the lumbosacral junction is usually needed as well. Oblique projections, sitting and bending views, or tomography may be useful in some instances. CT is valuable for detailed analysis of many spinal fractures (Fig. 3.15). For instance, it can clarify the anatomic derangements associated with spinal injuries, such as retropulsion (posterior displacement of fragments into the vertebral canal) and facet dislocations. It is especially useful for evaluating injuries of the lumbar spine, since it allows simultaneous visualization of the adjacent abdominal structures, which are often injured as well.

Among the common injuries to which the thoracic spine and the lumbosacral spine are subject are the following:

1. Simple compression fractures (Figs. 3.16, 3.17). Most traumatic thoracic fractures occur in the lower thoracic spine; fractures of the middle and upper thoracic spine are often secondary to underlying pathology, such as senile osteoporosis or metastatic tumor.
2. Fracture-dislocations (Fig. 3.18). A dislocation of one vertebra may be linked with a fracture of another.
3. Posterior element fractures (Figs. 3.19, 3.20). When these involve the transverse processes, they often represent avulsion fractures at the attachments of the psoas muscle.

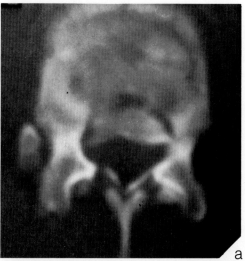

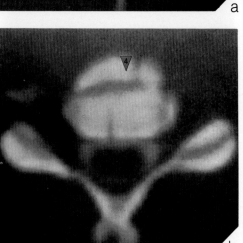

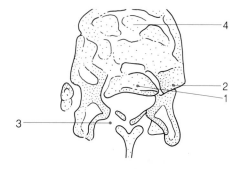

1	Posteriorly displaced portion of vertebral body	3	Fractures of lamina
2	Fracture of pedicle	4	Fractures of vertebral body

Fig. 3.15 Use of CT to evaluate spinal injuries. *a Axial CT scan accurately delineates the extent of this compression fracture. The body is comminuted; the posterior part of the vertebral body is retropulsed into the vertebral canal, and the left pedicle and both laminae are fractured. b In another patient, an axial CT scan obtained after injection of metrizamide into the subarachnoid space shows a transverse fracture of the vertebral body (arrow 4). There is no compression of the subarachnoid space or spinal cord edema.*

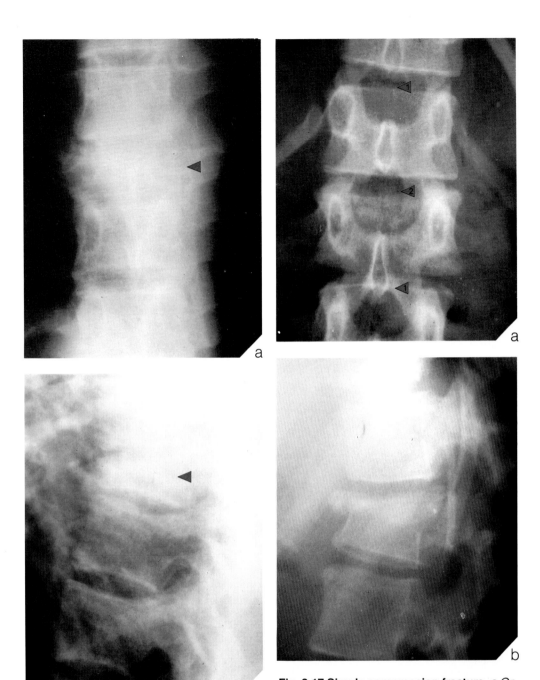

Fig. 3.16 Compression fracture. *a* Frontal and *b* lateral radiographs of the thoracic spine reveal loss of vertebral body height and wedging of T7 (arrows).

Fig. 3.17 Simple compression fracture. *a* On the frontal radiograph the end-plates of T11, T12, and L2 are well-defined and appear as continuous lines (arrows 1), but the superior end-plate of L1 (arrow 2) is not well seen. *b* The lateral view shows loss of vertebral body height and depression of the superior end-plate. Because of the deformity the x-ray beam is not tangent to the end-plate and therefore it is not visible on the frontal radiograph.

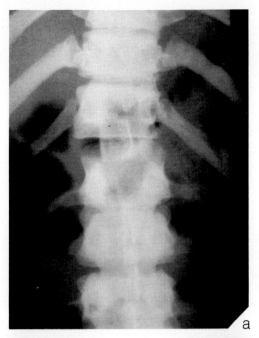

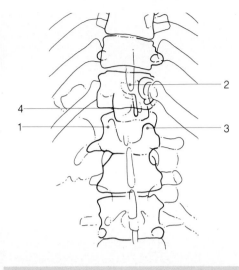

1	L1 vertebral body	3	Naked superior facet of L1
2	T12 vertebral body	4	Inferior facet of L1

Fig. 3.18 Fracture-dislocation of T12–L1.
*Frontal projection shows asymmetric narrowing of the T1–L1 disc space. In addition, the end-plates and the spinous process of L1 are not well visualized. The superior facets of L1 are "naked" and not articulate with the inferior facets of T12. **b** Lateral projection show anterior dislocation of T12 and a fracture of the superior end-plate of L1.*

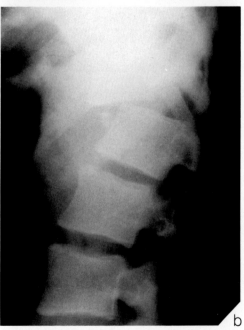

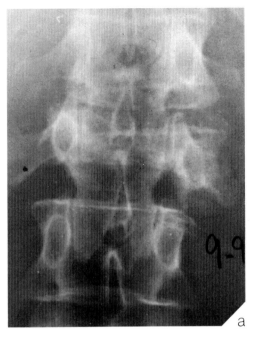

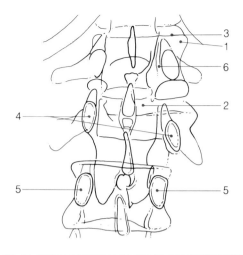

1	L1 vertebral body	4	L2 pedicles
2	L2 vertebral body	5	L3 pedicles
3	L1 superior endplate	6	L1 laminar fracture

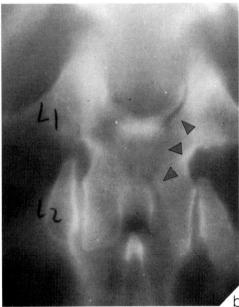

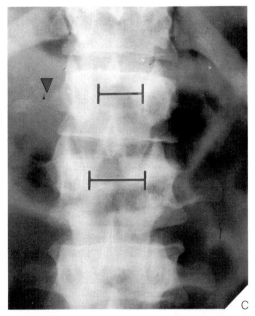

Fig. 3.19 Posterior element fractures. *These fractures are well seen on the frontal projection if the structures that normally overlap on this view are carefully evaluated.* ***a*** *A compression/ rotation injury of L2 is shown. The vertebral body is obviously disrupted and collapsed. The distance between the pedicles of L2 is increased (compare with L3 and L4). The upper spine (L2 and above) is displaced to the left with respect to the lower spine (L3 and below). Note the subtle fracture of the left lami-* na of L1: *Spinal fractures often are multiple and can only be detected by compulsive film reading.* ***b*** *A pluridirectional tomogram confirms the fracture of the L1 lamina (arrows).* ***c*** *In another patient, frontal projection shows a fracture line across the lamina and pedicle, widening of the interpedicular distance (bars), and a vertical split of the vertebral body. In addition, there is a fracture of the right transverse process of L1 (arrow).*

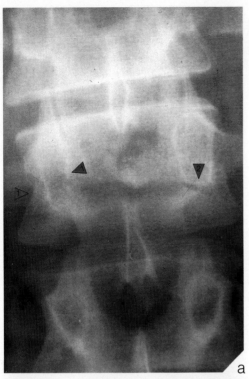

a

Fig. 3.20 Posterior element fractures.
a Frontal projection shows a fracture involving the pedicle on the right (arrows 1) *and the lamina on the left* (arrow 2) *b* Frontal projection in another patient shows fractures of the L3 and L4 transverse processes on the left (arrows).

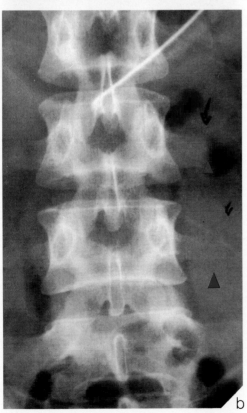

b

EXAMINATION OF THE SACRUM

Fractures of the sacrum are typically and frequently a major component of pelvic fractures. As a consequence, pelvic fractures may be accompanied by major retroperitoneal hemorrhage. Sacral alar fractures, the most common type of sacrum fracture, can be identified by discontinuity of the anterior superior sacral foraminal lines on a frontal view (Fig. 3.21). The less common transverse sacral fracture cannot be visualized on a frontal projection, but as is evident from Fig. 3.22, it is easily seen on a lateral projection.

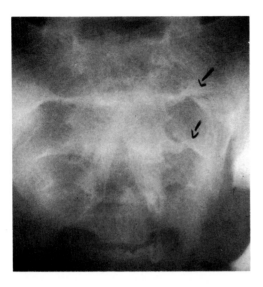

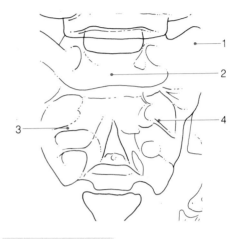

1 Sacral ala
2 Sacral body
  (S2 segment)
3 Normal anterior
  superior
  sacral foraminal
  line
4 Disrupted
  anterior
  superior
  sacral foraminal
  line

Fig. 3.21 Fracture of sacral ala. *Frontal projection of the sacrum shows discontinuity of the anterior superior sacra foraminal lines on the left. The normal line is seen on the right. These innocuous appearing fractures indicate major trauma and may be associated with life-threatening hemorrhage, and nerve root and parasympathetic injuries. They can result in impotence, frigidity, and urinary and fecal incontinence.*

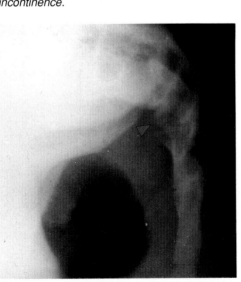

Fig. 3.22 Transverse sacral fracture. *Lateral projection shows a fracture through the upper sacrum (arrow). This fracture usually results from a fall on the buttocks. It can be reliably identified only on a lateral radiograph.*

Fractures and Dislocations of the Upper Extremity

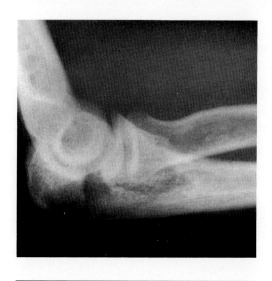

SHOULDER AND ARM INJURIES

The upper extremity extends from the shoulder to the distal phalanges of the fingers and is attached to the axial skeleton at the sternum (Fig. 4.1). Fractures of the clavicle are common and usually occur in the middle third of the bone (Fig. 4.2) or at the distal end near the acromioclavicular joint; fractures of the inner third are rare. Patients with midclavicular fractures should be carefully examined for concomitant fractures and dislocations of the upper ribs. Dislocation of the clavicle may occur at either the sternoclavicular or the acromioclavicular joint (Fig. 4.3).

Shoulder dislocations are the most common of all joint dislocations. In the usual type of shoulder dislocation, the humeral head is displaced anterior to the glenoid fossa. An impaction fracture of the posterolateral aspect of the humeral head (Hill-Sacks deformity) is often present, especially in patients with recurrent dislocations (Fig. 4.4). Posterior dislocations are less common and are easily missed (Fig. 4.5); other types of dislocation are rare. The proximal humerus and scapula should be carefully inspected in any patient with a shoulder dislocation, since associated fractures are quite common (Fig. 4.6; see also Fig. 4.4).

Fractures of the proximal humerus may occur alone or in association with a shoulder dislocation. Such fractures may involve (individually or in combination) the anatomic segment, the greater or lesser tuberosity, or the surgical neck (Fig. 4.7).

Humeral shaft fractures may be comminuted, oblique, transverse, or spiral (Fig. 4.8). When obtaining radiographs of patients with fractures of the proximal or mid humerus, the technologist must not rotate the patient's arm, for doing so may damage the artery or nerve or exacerbate an existing neurovascular injury.

Fractures of the distal humerus may be extraarticular (supracondylar, medial epicondylar, or lateral epicondylar) or intraarticular (transcondylar, condylar, capitellar, or trochlear) (Figs. 4.9–4.12).

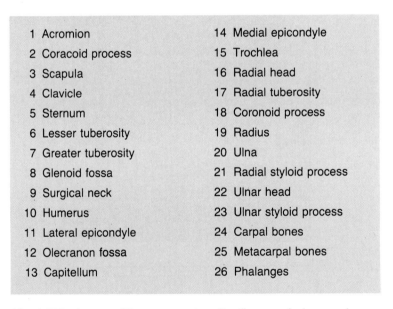

1 Acromion	14 Medial epicondyle
2 Coracoid process	15 Trochlea
3 Scapula	16 Radial head
4 Clavicle	17 Radial tuberosity
5 Sternum	18 Coronoid process
6 Lesser tuberosity	19 Radius
7 Greater tuberosity	20 Ulna
8 Glenoid fossa	21 Radial styloid process
9 Surgical neck	22 Ulnar head
10 Humerus	23 Ulnar styloid process
11 Lateral epicondyle	24 Carpal bones
12 Olecranon fossa	25 Metacarpal bones
13 Capitellum	26 Phalanges

Fig. 4.1 The bones of the upper extremity *(figure on facing page).*

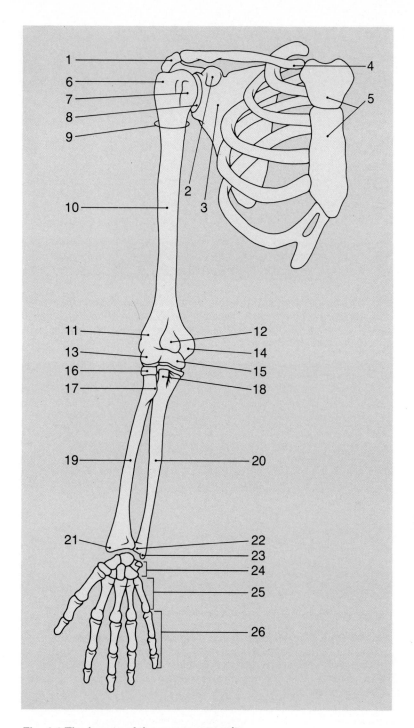

Fig. 4.1 The bones of the upper extremity.

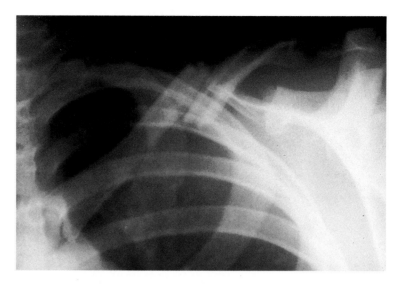

Fig. 4.2 Clavicular shaft fracture. *Frontal projection shows a fracture of the middle part of the clavicle, the most common type of clavicular fracture. The medial fragment, which is attached to the sternocleidomastoid muscle, is displaced upward.*

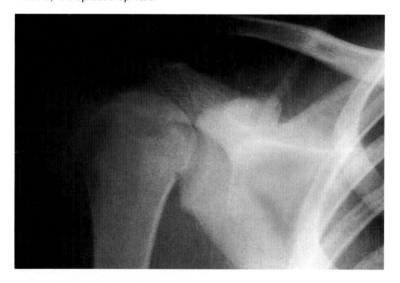

Fig. 4.3 Type III acromioclavicular dislocation. *Frontal projection shows wide separation of the acromion and coracoid from the clavicle, indicating disruption of the acromioclavicular and coracoclavicular ligaments. Weight-bearing views may be necessary to distinguish a sprain from a complete tear.*

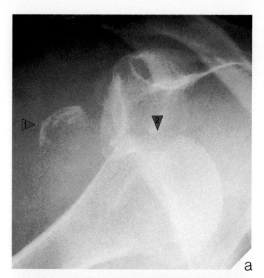

Fig. 4.4 Subcoracoid anterior dislocation of the shoulder. *a* Frontal view shows the humeral head displaced under the coracoid process. There is a displaced fracture of the greater tuberosity (arrow 1). *Note defect (arrow 2) in the posterolateral aspect of the humeral head (Hill-Sacks deformity). **b*** On the posterior oblique "Y" projection, the humeral head is projected anterior to the glenoid fossa. The "Y" view is essential for evaluating shoulder trauma.

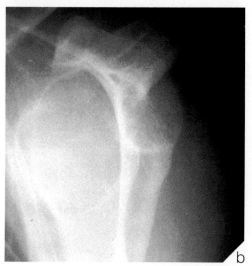

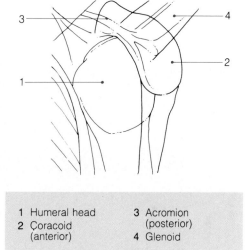

1 Humeral head	3 Acromion
2 Coracoid	(posterior)
(anterior)	4 Glenoid

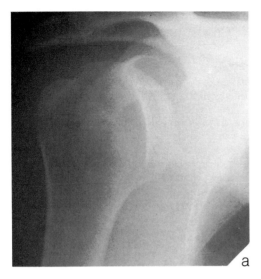
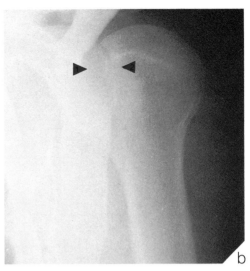

Fig. 4.5 Posterior dislocation of the shoulder. *a Anterior oblique view shows the humeral head superimposed on the glenoid. **b** On the posterior oblique view, the humeral head* (arrow 1) *lies posterior to the glenoid fossa impacted on the posterior lip of the glenoid* (arrow 2).

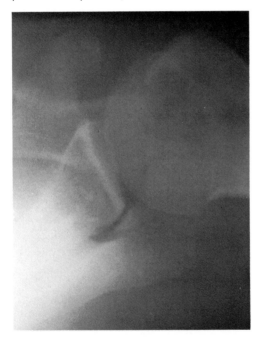

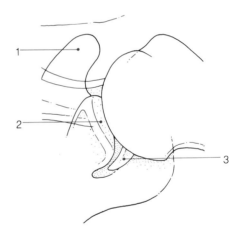

Fig. 4.6 Shoulder dislocation with fracture of glenoid. *Axillary projection of the shoulder shows a small fracture of the posterior glenoid caused by avulsion of the glenoid labrum. When an anterior or posterior dislocation has been diagnosed, the axillary projection should be obtained to evaluate the glenoid and the humeral head.*

1 Acromion	3 Fracture of the posterior glenoid
2 Glenoid	

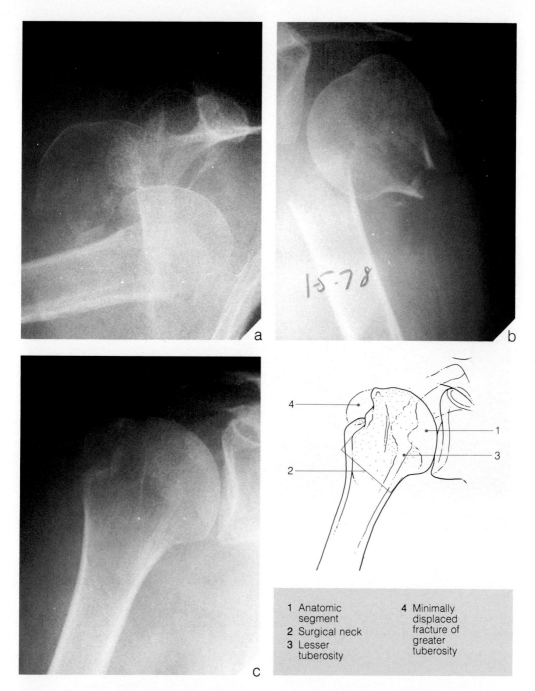

1	Anatomic segment	4	Minimally displaced fracture of greater tuberosity
2	Surgical neck		
3	Lesser tuberosity		

Fig. 4.7 Fractures of the proximal humerus.
a Four-part fracture-dislocation of the proximal humerus. Fractures of the anatomic segment and the surgical neck can be seen on this view. Fractures of both tuberosities were seen on other projections. *b* Transverse displaced frac- ture of the humerus is evident. The shaft is displaced medially by the pull of the pectoralis major muscle. *c* A minimally displaced fracture of the greater tuberosity of the humerus can be seen; other structures are normal.

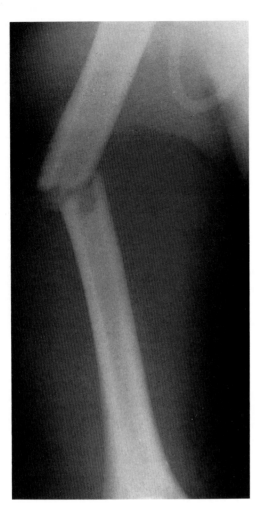

Fig. 4.8 Transverse fracture of the humeral shaft. *Rotational views of the shoulder are contraindicated in this type of fracture since inadvertent movement of the fragments may cause an iatrogenic neurovascular injury. A transthoracic lateral projection is preferred as the "second view" in any patient with a suspected fracture of the humerus.*

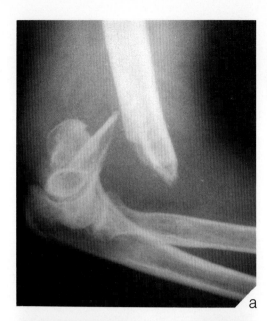

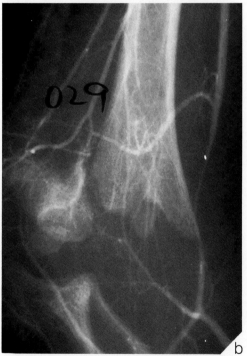

Fig. 4.9 Supracondylar fractures. *a In the extension-type supracondylar fracture of the distal humerus shown here, brachial artery injury is an important potential complication. Arteriography should be performed if the pulses are diminished. b A brachial arteriogram in another patient with a supracondylar fracture shows marked spasm but no occlusion or bleeding.*

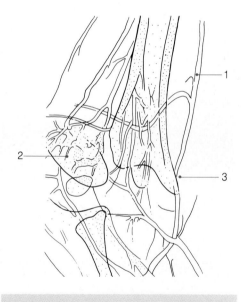

1	Brachial artery	3 Area of brachial artery narrowing
2	Displaced humoral condyle	

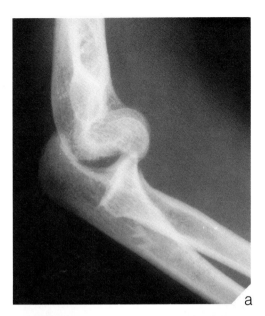

a

Fig. 4.10 Distal humeral fracture. *a* *On the lateral projection, the capitellum of the humerus is fractured, rotated, and displaced anteriorly. **b** The anteroposterior projection shows superimposition of the capitellar fragments.*

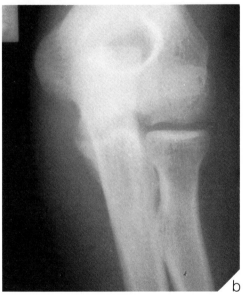

b

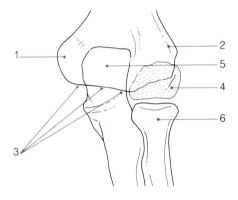

1 Medial	4 Capitellar
epicondyle	fragment
2 Lateral	5 Olecranon
epicondyle	process
3 Trochlea	6 Radial head

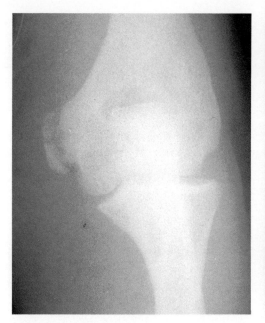

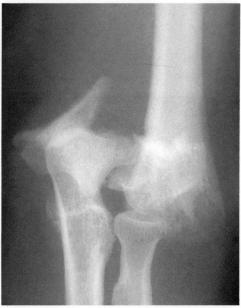

Fig. 4.11 Avulsion of medial epicondyle.
Frontal projection shows avulsion of the ununited medial epicondyle in a teenager who was hit by a car while walking. This injury results from violent contraction of the forearm flexors, which originate on the medial epicondyle. Pitching a baseball can produce partial or complete avulsion of the medial epicondyle in children and adolescents ("little league elbow").

Fig. 4.12 Intercondylar fracture of the humerus. *The medial and lateral fragments are displaced apart and angulated inward by the pull of the flexors and extensors of the forearm.*

ELBOW AND FOREARM INJURIES

The elbow is a complex joint composed of three articulations: the radiohumeral, the ulnohumeral, and the radioulnar. Although dislocation of any one of these articulations may occur in isolation, the most commonly seen injury is combined radiohumeral-ulnohumeral dislocation (Fig. 4.13). Elbow dislocations may be associated with fractures of the radial head or neck, of the coronoid or olecranon processes of the ulna, or of the distal humerus. Intra- and periarticular fractures may also occur as isolated injuries (Figs. 4.14, 4.15).

One must remember that since the forearm bones join at their proximal and distal ends to form a rectangle, it is difficult to break or displace a single forearm bone without causing a fracture or dislocation in another part of the rectangle (Fig. 4.16a). For example, in the Galeazzi fracture a fracture of the distal shaft of the radius is accompanied by a dislocation of the distal radioulnar joint (Fig. 4.16b); and in the Monteggia fracture, a fracture of the proximal shaft of the ulna is associated with a dislocation of the proximal radioulnar joint (Fig. 4.16). Thus, when an isolated forearm fracture is seen, one should assume the presence of another injury until this is definitely excluded.

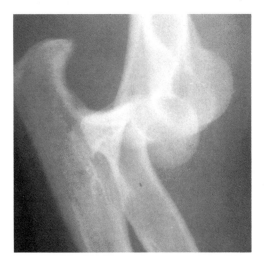

Fig. 4.13 Posterior dislocation of the elbow. *The radius and the ulna are dislocated as a unit. Posterior and posterolateral dislocations are the most common.*

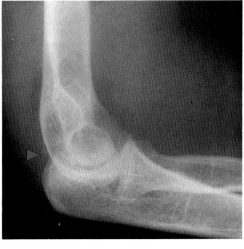

Fig. 4.14 Positive fat pad sign. *Lateral projection of the elbow shows elevation of the posterior fat pad (arrow), indicating the presence of intraarticular fluid (blood). Other projections demonstrated a subtle undisplaced fracture of the radial head.*

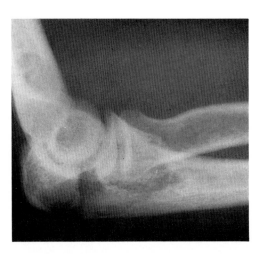

Fig. 4.15 Olecranon fracture. *Lateral projection shows a fracture through the olecranon process. The proximal fragment is displaced proximally as a result of the pull of the triceps muscle.*

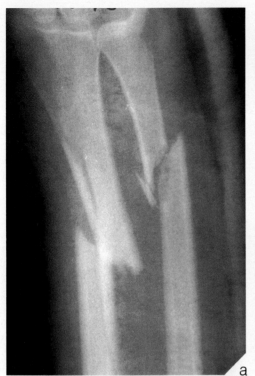

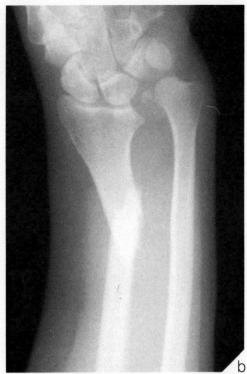

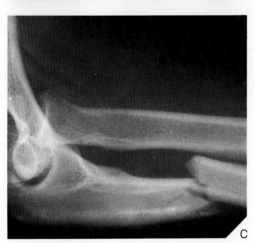

Fig. 4.16 Forearm fractures. *a Double-bone forearm fracture. b Galeazzi fracture: The distal radial shaft is fractured, and the distal radioulnar joint is disrupted. c Monteggia fracture: The proximal ulnar shaft is fractured, with anterior displacement and posterior angulation of the distal fragment. (Alternatively this could be described as "anterior angulation of the fracture apex.") There is anterior dislocation of the radial head.*

WRIST AND HAND INJURIES

The wrist is composed of eight carpal bones arranged in two rows. The proximal row articulates with the radius (directly) and the ulna (indirectly); the distal row articulates with the metacarpal bones. The hand consists of the carpal bones of the wrist, the five metacarpals, and the five proximal, five middle, and five distal phalanges (Figs. 4.17, 4.18). Fractures and dislocations of the wrist and hand are the most common type of skeletal injury.

The Colles fracture consists of (1) a dorsally displaced, distal radial metaphyseal fracture that may involve the distal radioulnar or the radiocarpal joints and (2) a fracture of the ulnar styloid process (Fig. 4.19a,b). The Smith fracture is associated with volar displacement of the distal radial fragment (Fig. 4.19c). It must be distinguished from the Colles fracture, for the two injuries require opposite approaches to reduction and casting.

Fracture of the scaphoid (navicula) is the most common fracture of the carpal bones (Fig. 4.20). Navicular fractures are often subtle; in some instances, they may even be invisible on the initial radiographic examination. Because of the risk of nonunion, it is best to immobilize the wrist if clinical findings suggest a fracture, and then to repeat the films, with the cast removed, two weeks later. Radionuclide scintigraphy also can be used to confirm or exclude the presence of a fracture.

Carpal dislocations usually are perilunar. Perilunar dislocations are best seen on the lateral projection, which shows a normal relation between the lunate and the articular surface of the radius, but dorsal displacement of the remaining carpal bones (Fig. 4.21). Associated fractures of the scaphoid, triquetrum, capitate, or radius may be present.

Occupational and sports injuries of the hand are common, especially avulsions and fingertip crush injuries (Fig. 4.22a). Avulsion fractures of the phalanges occur at the attachments of ligaments and tendons, particularly at the dorsal aspect of the articular surface of the distal phalanx (mallet finger; Fig. 4.22b). Phalangeal shaft fractures may be spiral, transverse, oblique, or intraarticular. Metacarpal fractures usually involve the fifth metacarpal bone (boxer's fracture) or the first metacarpal bone (Bennett and Rolando fractures) (Fig. 4.22c).

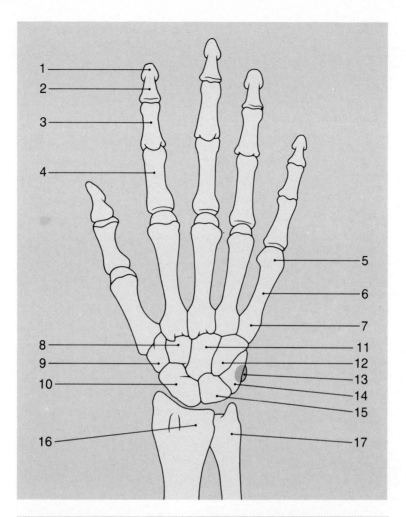

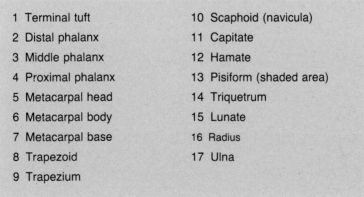

1 Terminal tuft	10 Scaphoid (navicula)
2 Distal phalanx	11 Capitate
3 Middle phalanx	12 Hamate
4 Proximal phalanx	13 Pisiform (shaded area)
5 Metacarpal head	14 Triquetrum
6 Metacarpal body	15 Lunate
7 Metacarpal base	16 Radius
8 Trapezoid	17 Ulna
9 Trapezium	

Fig. 4.17 Dorsal view of the hand and wrist.

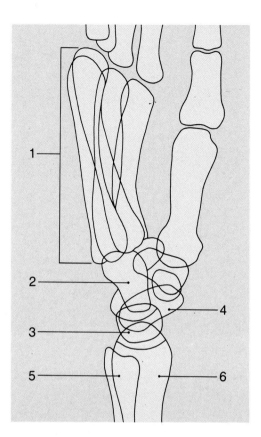

Fig. 4.18 Lateral view of the wrist showing normal anatomy.

1 metacarpal bones   4 ulna
2 capitate   5 radius
3 lunate

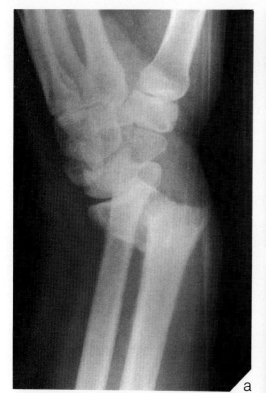

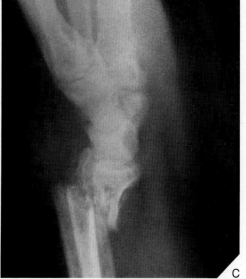

Fig. 4.19 Wrist fractures. *a, b* In a Colles fracture, the distal radial metaphysis is displaced and angulated dorsally on the lateral projection (*b*). Associated injuries (not seen here) may include fractures of the ulnar styloid process and scaphoid (navicula). *c* A lateral radiograph of a Smith fracture shows anterior displacement and anterior angulation of the distal radius. The angulation of the distal fragment is opposite to that of a Colles fracture.

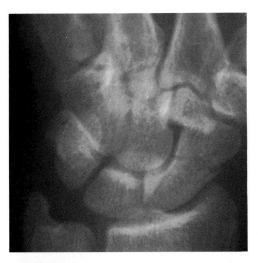

Fig. 4.20 Scaphoid fracture. Fractures such as this one through the middle of the scaphoid are common carpal injuries. Nonunion and avascular necrosis are frequent complications.

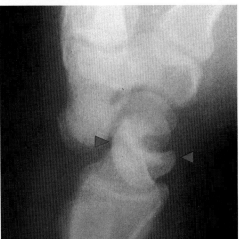

Fig. 4.21 Perilunar dislocation. *A lateral radiograph shows the lunate* (arrows) *sitting in a normal fashion on the articular surface of the radius, but the remaining carpal bones are displaced dorsally.*

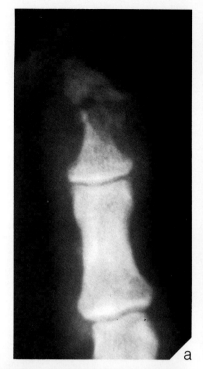
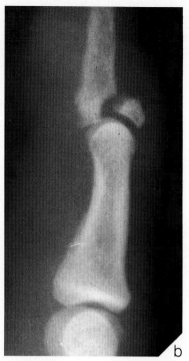

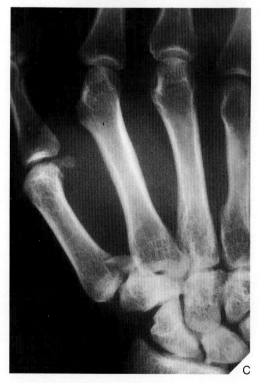

Fig. 4.22 Hand fractures. *a* *In this eggshell fracture, the terminal tuft of the finger has been crushed. Such injuries usually result from slamming a finger in a door.* ***b*** *The fragment seen is this radiograph of a mallet finger is the attachment of the extensor tendon of the finger.* ***c*** *A Bennett's fracture is an intraarticular avulsion fracture of the base of the 1st (thumb) metacarpal. It is nearly always unstable because of the unopposed pull of the abductor pollicis longus and abductor pollicis muscles.*

C H A P T E R   F I V E

Fractures of the Pelvis

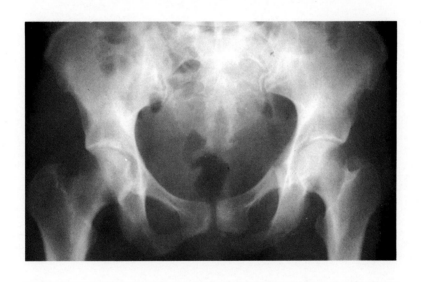

Pelvic fractures are common, ranging from minor sports-related fractures to major injuries (usually caused by a motor vehicle accident or a fall from a height). Major pelvic fractures are frequently associated with massive hemorrhage and are among the leading causes of death from trauma.

The pelvis joins the lower extremities to the axial skeleton. It is composed of two innominate bones that are joined to each other anteriorly and to the sacrum posteriorly (Fig. 5.1). This arrangement allows weight to be distributed up the lower extremities, through the acetabula, and across the sacroiliac joints to the spine.

AVULSION FRACTURES

Avulsion fractures occur when a muscle contracts with a force that is sufficient to detach its bony insertion. These fractures occur commonly in association with sports such as hurdling or broad jumping. There are three common types of avulsion fractures (Fig. 5.2): (1) avulsion of the anterosuperior iliac spine by the sartorius muscle; (2) avulsion of the anteroinferior iliac spine by the rectus femoris muscle (Fig. 5.3); and (3) avulsion of the ischial tuberosity by the adductor muscles (Fig. 5.4). The degree of displacement determines how the injury will be treated, and therefore should be carefully assessed on the films. Radiographs obtained during the healing phase can be confusing, because exuberant bone production can mimic osteogenic sarcoma (see Fig. 5.4a).

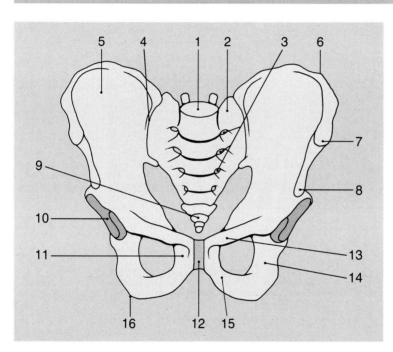

Fig. 5.1 Anatomic diagram of the pelvis.

1 Body of sacrum	9 Coccyx
2 Ala of sacrum	10 Acetabulum
3 Anterior sacral foramina	11 Body of pubis
4 Sacroiliac joint	12 Symphysis pubis
5 Ilium	13 Superior pubic ramus
6 Iliac crest	14 Ramus of ischium
7 Anterosuperior iliac spine	15 Inferior pubic ramus
8 Anteroinferior iliac spine	16 Ischial tuberosity

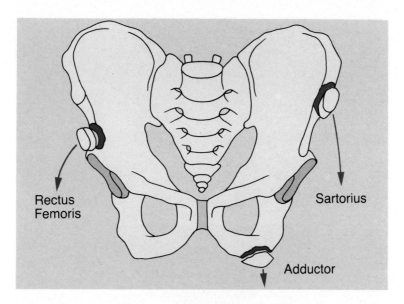

Fig. 5.2 Avulsion fractures: sartorius, adductor, and rectus femoris.

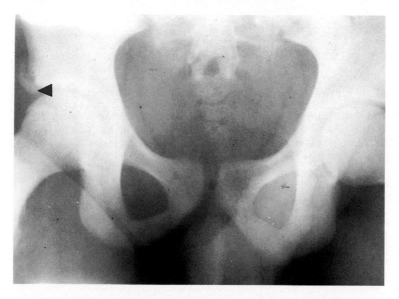

Fig. 5.3 Avulsion fracture. *Anteroposterior projection shows an undisplaced avulsion fracture of the right anteroinferior iliac spine* (arrow).

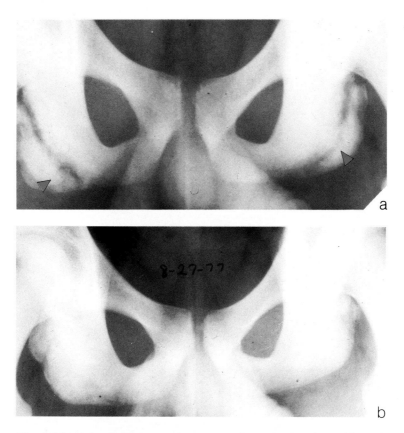

Fig. 5.4 Avulsion fractures. *a Anteroposterior projection shows bilateral ischial tuberosity avulsion fractures* (arrows) *in a teenage hurdler. There is a considerable new bone production at both fracture sites, indicating that the fractures are several weeks old.* **b** *One year later, both fractures have healed.*

SINGLE BONE FRACTURES

In a single bone fracture (Fig. 5.5), the mechanism of injury is a single direct blow to the fracture site. On the whole, such fractures are unusual. The most common fractures of this type are fractures of the iliac wing (Duverney fractures; Fig. 5.6a), transverse sacral fractures (Fig. 5.6b), and isolated pubic rami fractures (Fig. 5.7). Transverse sacral fractures result from a fall on the buttocks. The fracture often cannot be detected on the frontal projection; it may go undiagnosed unless a lateral radiograph is obtained (see Figs. 5.6b, 3.22). Bed rest usually is sufficient treatment for single bone fractures, which generally do not affect weight-bearing.

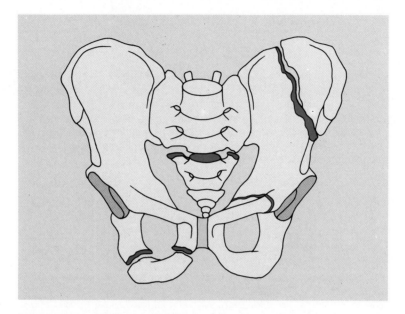

Fig. 5.5 Single bone fractures.

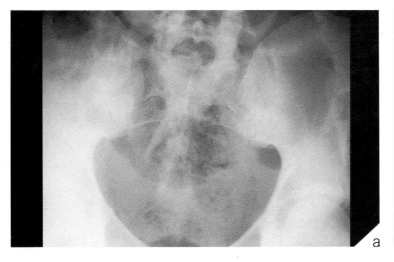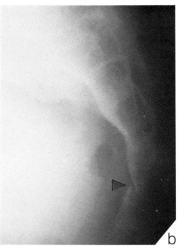

Fig. 5.6 Single bone fractures. *a This isolated comminuted fracture of the left iliac wing (Duverney fracture) resulted from a direct blow to the ilium. b Lateral radiograph of the sacrum shows an isolated horizontal fracture of the sacral cortex* (arrow) *caused by a direct impact from a fall. Such fractures are frequently invisible on frontal projections.*

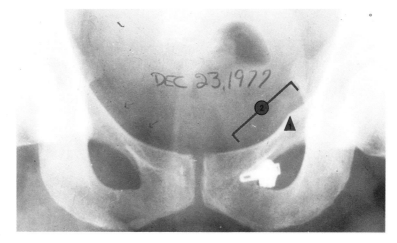

Fig. 5.7 Single bone fracture of the pubis. *Anteroposterior projection shows an isolated undisplaced fracture of the left superior pubic ramus. Note the subtle buckling of the cortex* (arrow 1) *and the loss of obturator fat plane* (brace 2) *on the side of the fracture.*

MULTIPLE BONE FRACTURES

The pelvis may be thought of as a series of rings, two minor and one major. The two minor rings are formed by the ischium and pubis on each side. The posterior half of the major ring is formed by the iliac wings, the sacroiliac joints, and the sacrum; the anterior half is formed by the two minor rings, which are joined at the symphysis pubis.

Together, the pelvic rings form a complex structure that somewhat resembles a pretzel. The analogy is apt: For much the same reasons that it is almost impossible to break a pretzel in only one place, it is difficult to fracture the pelvis in only one spot. Major pelvic injuries usually cause multiple fractures; therefore, single breaks should be viewed with suspicion.

Minor Ring Fractures

Minor ring fractures typically take the form of breaks of the anterior portion of the greater ring (Fig. 5.8). A second fracture (or dislocation) is commonly found in the posterior portion of the major ring (Figs. 5.9, 5.10; see Major Ring Fractures, below). The most common of these pelvic injuries are the following:

1. Sacroiliac dislocation. The sacroiliac joints are normally symmetrical, with the inner margin of the ilium usually meeting the second sacral foraminal line. Sacroiliac dislocation is indicated by a widening of the joint space or by elevation of the iliac line in relation to the sacral line.
2. Sacral fractures. The anterosuperior sacral foraminal lines are the key to diagnosing sacral fractures. Normally, the first and second sacral foraminal lines appear as smooth, single, uniform crescentic densities. Fractures disrupt these lines, making them invisible, jagged, buckled, or discontinuous.

3. Iliac fractures. Iliac wing fractures typically follow a vertical oblique course. They are often subtle. The fracture line may be obscured by overlying bowel gas, or the fragments may overlap in such a way that the fracture line is not seen. If one follows the cortex of the iliac crest, the fracture will usually become apparent.

A direct blow to the pubic arch may result in disruption of the pubic symphysis (Fig. 5.11) or multiple fractures of the pubic rami (Fig. 5.12). Fractures of the pubic rami can often be effectively evaluated through use of CT (Fig. 5.13).

Major Ring Fractures

Major ring (Malgaigne) fractures are combinations of minor ring breaks and posterior element fractures (Figs. 5.14–5.16). Double ring fractures, which are often associated with massive hemorrhage and pelvic instability, are the most serious of these; sometimes they are lethal. Complications include sexual dysfunction, urinary retention, fecal incontinence, chronic low back pain, limb shortening, and limp.

CT is useful in evaluating major ring fractures because it displays anterior and posterior structures without superimposition and because it adds the important axial plane to the perspective provided by conventional radiographs. It is especially helpful in the assessment of iliac wing fractures (Figs. 5.17, 5.18), sacral alar fractures (Fig. 5.19), and sacroiliac dislocation (Fig. 5.20). In addition, it is of particular value in the diagnosis and management of acetabular fractures (see Acetabular Fractures, below). CT can also demonstrate the retroperitoneal hemorrhage and lower urinary tract injuries that are often associated with pelvic fractures.

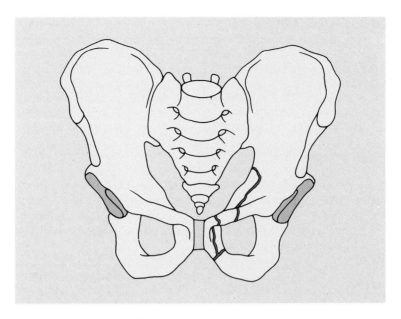

Fig. 5.8 Minor ring fractures.

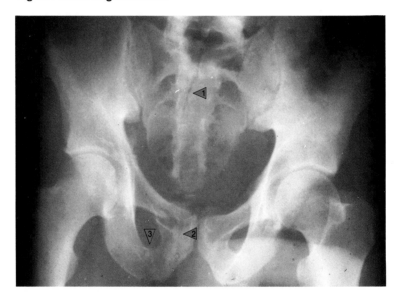

Fig. 5.9 Major ring fracture. *Anteroposterior projection shows a vertical fracture of the body of the sacrum (arrow 1) and fractures of the body (arrow 2) and the inferior ramus (arrow 3) of the pubis. The sacral fracture could be seen only on the frontal projection.*

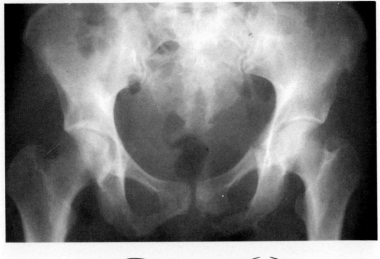

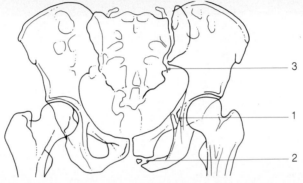

1 Fracture of the superior
  pubic ramus
2 Fracture of the inferior
  pubic ramus

3 Fracture of the sacral ala

Fig. 5.10 Major ring fracture. *Anteroposterior projection shows a double pubic fracture on the left: one in the superior pubic ramus near the acetabulum, the other through the inferior pubic ramus. Since it is unusual to encounter this combination as an isolated injury, the remainder of the pelvis should be carefully scrutinized for additional fractures. In this patient there is also a fracture of the left sacral ala.*

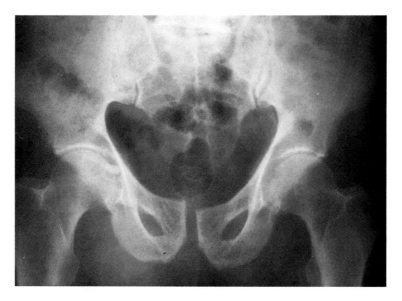

Fig. 5.11 Disruption of symphysis pubis. *Note asymmetry of the symphysis pubis as a result of disruption of the ligamentous support.*

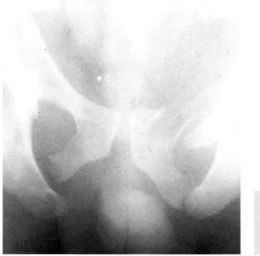

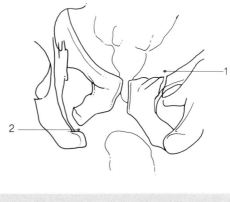

| 1 Fracture of the superior pubic ramus | 2 Fracture of the inferior pubic ramus |

Fig. 5.12 Straddle fracture of pubic arch. *Anteroposterior shows bilateral fractures of the superior and inferior pubic rami. Such fractures are usually due to a fall from a height.*

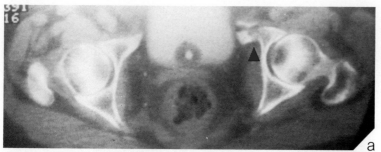
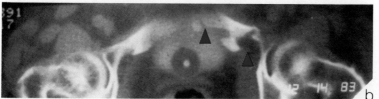
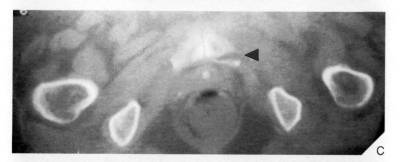
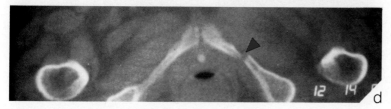

Fig. 5.13 Minor ring fractures.
*CT scans of the pubic arch. **a** A cut at the level of the superior pubic rami shows a comminuted fracture of the left superior pubic ramus (arrow). **b** A slightly more caudal cut shows a fracture through the body of the left pubis (left arrow). The fracture of the superior pubic ramus (right arrow) is again seen. **c** A cut at the level of the obturator ring shows the fracture through the body of the pubis (arrow). **d** A more caudal cut shows a fracture of the left inferior pubic ramus (arrow).*

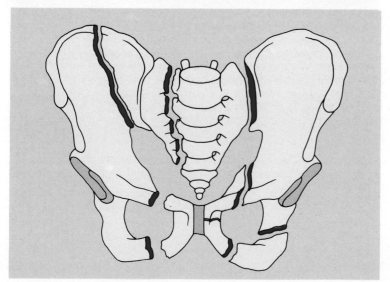

Fig. 5.14 Major ring (Malgaigne) fractures and dislocations.

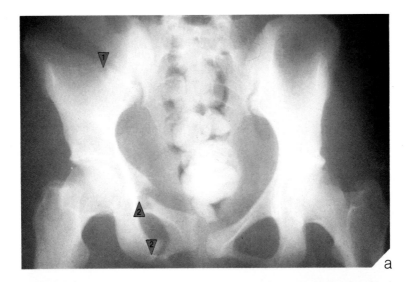

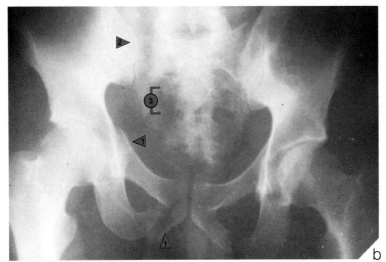

Fig. 5.15 Major ring (Malgaigne) fractures. *Radiographs of four patients show variants of the major ring (Malgaigne) fracture, an injury complex in which one hip is separated from the rest of the pelvis. **a** Iliac Malgaigne fracture. There are fractures through the right iliac wing (arrow 1) and the right pubic rami (arrows 2), isolating the right hip from the rest of the pelvis. Note the superior elevation of the right hip caused by unopposed muscle pull. **b** Sacral Malgaigne fracture. There are double pubic rami fractures on the right (arrows 1) as well as a subtle sacral fracture (arrow 2). In addition, there is discontinuity of the anterosuperior forami-*

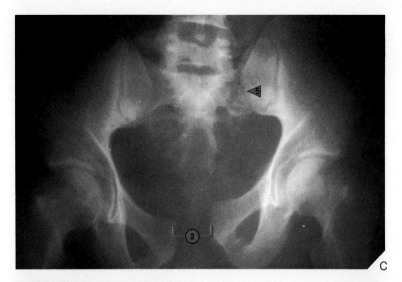

c

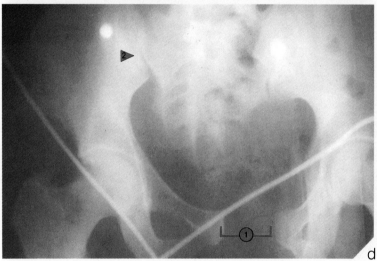

d

nal lines (brace 3), *indicating a fracture of the sacral ala. Associated nerve damage may result in sexual dysfunction (impotence or frigidity).*
c *Sacral Malgaigne fracture. In this patient there is a fracture of the left sacral ala (arrow 5)* *and diastasis of the symphysis pubis (brace 2), isolating the left hip, which is elevated as a result of unopposed muscle pull.*
d *Innominate dislocation. Note the wide diastasis of the symphysis pubis (brace 1), right sacroiliac dislocation (arrow 2), and superior elevation of the right innominate bone.*

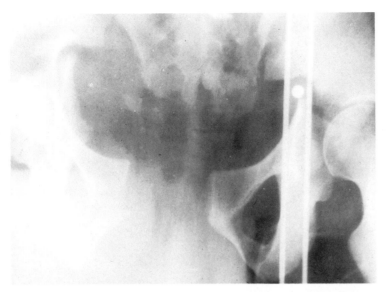

Fig. 5.16 Bilateral Malgaigne fracture ("crushed pelvis").
Anteroposterior projection shows a severely crushed pelvis resulting from a brick wall falling on the patient. Fractures of both acetabula, dislocation of both sacroiliac joints, dislocation of the symphysis pubis, and multiple fractures of the rami can be seen.

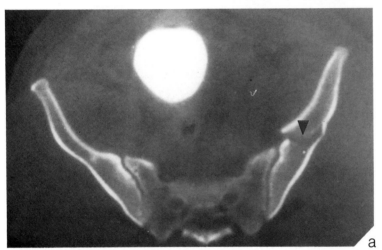

Fig. 5.17 Iliac wing fracture.
a CT scan shows a fracture through the left iliac wing (arrow). b A more caudal cut shows that the fracture extends into the acetabulum.

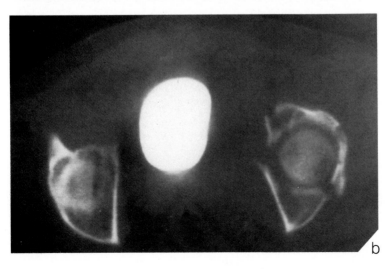

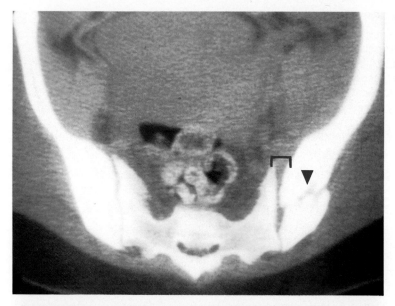

Fig. 5.18 Iliac wing fracture involving the sacroiliac joint. *CT scan shows a transverse fracture of the left ilium (arrow) extending into a diastatic sacroiliac joint (brace).*

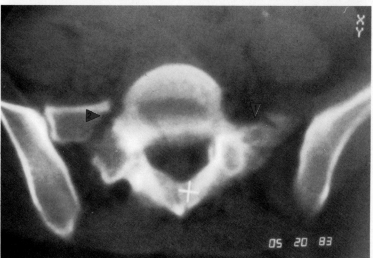

Fig. 5.19 Fractures of sacral alae. *CT scan demonstrates fractures through the left (arrow 1) and right (arrow 2) sacral alae above the level of the sacroiliac joint (arrow 1).*

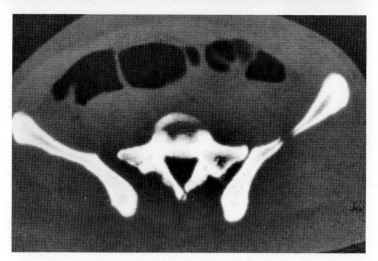

Fig. 5.20 Sacroiliac dislocation with iliac wing fracture. *CT scan shows right sacroiliac dislocation and a left iliac wing fracture.*

ACETABULAR FRACTURES

Acetabular fractures (Fig. 5.21) may be isolated (Fig. 5.22), associated with minor pelvic fractures (Fig. 5.23), or associated with a major ring fracture. Acetabular fractures are often caused by dislocation of the hip, either a posterior dislocation (Fig. 5.24), which may have reduced spontaneously, or a central hip dislocation. The latter results in an implosion fracture of the acetabulum with protrusion of the femoral head into the true pelvis (Fig. 5.25). Whereas implosion fractures are easily detected on the anteroposterior projection, posterior lip fractures may be difficult to see: Absence of a sharp posterior lip density may be the only clue on the frontal projection (Fig. 5.26a). Oblique views (Fig. 5.26b) and CT (Fig. 5.27) should be liberally employed in patients with suspected acetabular fractures. Intraarticular fragments, which must be surgically removed, are best visualized with CT (see Fig. 5.27b).

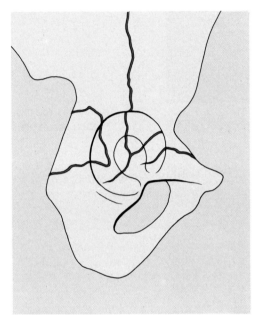

Fig. 5.21 Fractures of the acetabulum.

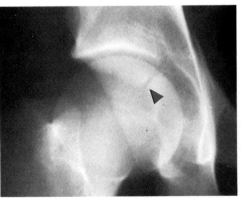

Fig. 5.22 Anterior acetabular fracture.
Anteroposterior projection of the hip shows an undisplaced fracture of the anterior portion of the acetabulum (arrow). The fracture does not extend into the posterior portion of the acetabulum.

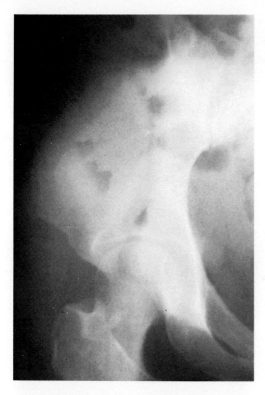

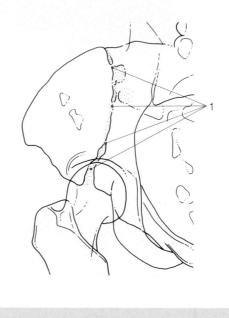

Fig. 5.23 Iliac fracture extending into acetabulum. *Anteroposterior projection shows* *a vertical fracture through the right ilium that extends into the roof of the acetabulum.*

Fig. 5.24 Hip dislocation with posterior acetabular fracture. *Anteroposterior projection of the hip shows complete posterior dislocation of the femoral head with a displaced posterior acetabular fragment.*

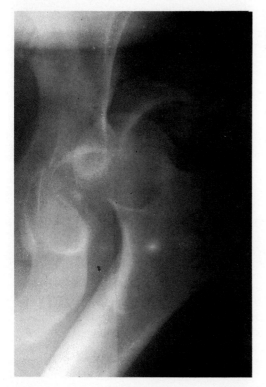

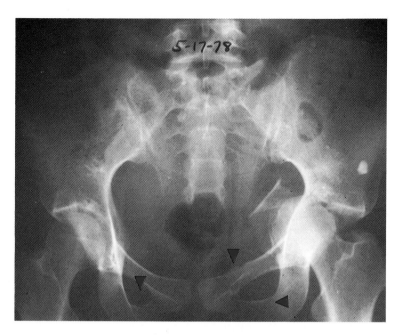

Fig. 5.25 Central hip dislocation. *Anteroposterior projection shows an implosion fracture of the central portion of the acetabulum with displacement of the femur into the true pelvis. Bilateral fractures of the pubic rami* (arrows) *can be seen.*

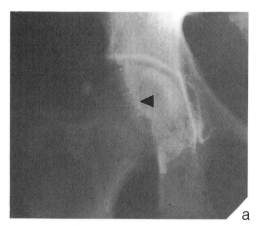

a

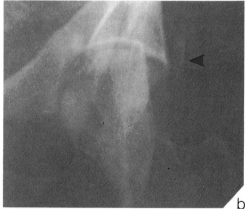

b

Fig. 5.26 Posterior acetabular fracture.
*a Anteroposterior projection shows a slightly displaced fracture of the posterior portion of the acetabulum (arrow). Although the fracture line is not easily discerned, the absence of the normal contour of the acetabular margin indicates the presence of a fracture. **b** The fracture fragment (arrow) is clearly seen on the oblique projection. Fractures of the posterior acetabulum are commonly associated with posterior hip dislocations, which often reduce spontaneously.*

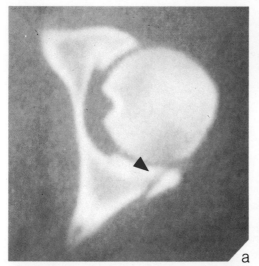

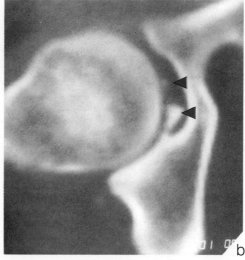

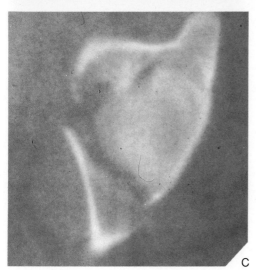

Fig. 5.27 Acetabular fractures. *a* CT scan shows an undisplaced posterior lip fracture (arrow). *b* In another patient, intraarticular fracture fragments (arrows) *can be seen adjacent to femoral head. Such fragments must be surgically removed.* *c* In a third patient, a comminuted fracture extends through the weight bearing portions of the acetabulum.

CHAPTER SIX

*F*ractures of the
Lower Extremity

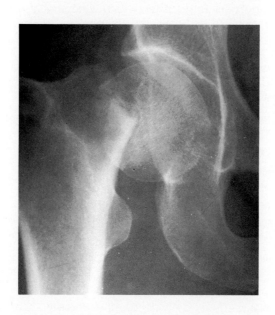

HIP AND THIGH FRACTURES

The lower extremity extends from the hip joint to the distal phalanges of the toes. It is attached to the axial skeleton at the pelvis, where the femoral head articulates with the acetabulum (Fig. 6.1). Acetabular fractures are often caused by hip dislocations, which though not rare, are much less common than shoulder dislocations. Hip dislocations are usually posterior, and therefore may be associated with fractures of the posterior acetabulum (Fig. 6.2). CT should be performed either before or after the dislocation is reduced (see Chapter Five); it is of considerable value in assessing the status of the acetabulum.

Fractures of the proximal femur can be impacted or nonimpacted, displaced or nondisplaced, simple or comminuted, stable or unstable. They may be difficult to recognize, especially when impacted; radionuclide scintigraphy and tomography can be useful diagnostic aids when questionable fracture lines are seen or when pain persists. These fractures of the proximal femur are in fact very common, often resulting from minor trauma in individuals with osteoporosis (e.g., postmenopausal women, elderly persons, and patients receiving corticosteroid therapy) (Figs. 6.3, 6.4). The distally based blood supply to the femoral head can be disrupted by an intracapsular fracture, and this disruption can lead to avascular necrosis. Avascular necrosis is most frequently associated with the uncommon segmental fracture of the femoral head. In general, the more distal the fracture, the smaller the risk of this sequela; in other words, avascular necrosis is more common after subcapital fracture than after midneck fracture, and least common after basicervical fractures.

Intertrochanteric fractures are extracapsular. The intertrochanteric region has an abundant blood supply, and even extensively comminuted fractures generally heal promptly. When evaluating an intertrochanteric fracture, one must determine whether the fracture line is single or comminuted; whether it involves the weight-bearing medial cortex (calcar); and whether displacement or impaction is present (Fig. 6.5). Isolated avulsion fractures of the trochanters are infrequent (Fig. 6.6). As a rule, the degree of displacement determines what form treatment takes. A subtrochanteric fracture can be considered either an extension of an intertrochanteric fracture or a high femoral shaft fracture (Fig. 6.7).

Femoral shaft fractures are usually obvious and easy to demonstrate radiographically (Fig. 6.8). One should not, how ever, be distracted by the obvious injury to the point where one misses the additional injuries that are often present. A thorough radiologic evaluation, including adequate views of the hip and knee, is essential. Shaft fractures are not uncommon after total hip replacement (Fig. 6.9).

1 Head of femur	12 Lateral condyle
2 Greater trochanter	13 Head of fibula
3 Intertrochanteric line	14 Neck
4 Lesser trochanter	15 Adductor tubercle
5 Symphysis pubis	16 Medial epicondyle
6 Pubic arch	17 Medial condyle
7 Obturator foramen	18 Tibial spines (anterior
8 Ischial tuberosity	and posterior)
9 Femur	19 Tuberosity
10 Patella	20 Fibula
11 Lateral epicondyle	21 Tibia

Fig. 6.1 Bones and joints of the lower extremity *(figure on facing page)*.

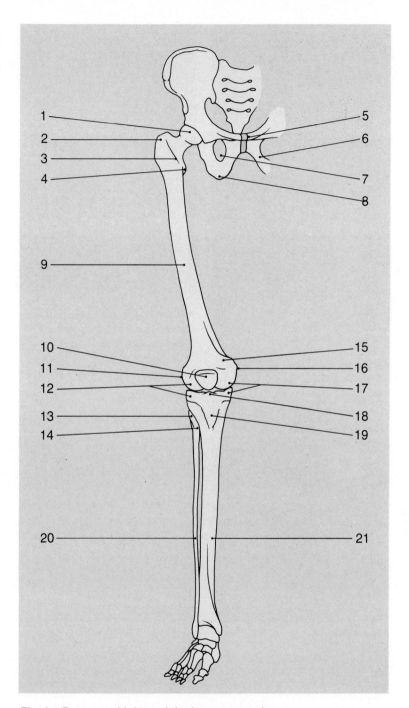

Fig. 6.1 Bones and joints of the lower extremity.

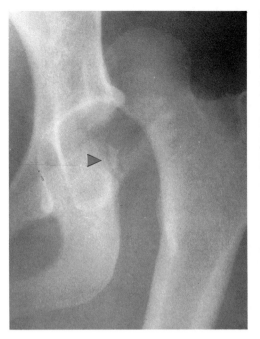

Fig. 6.2 Posterior hip dislocation. *Note the fragment of the posterior acetabulum* (arrow).

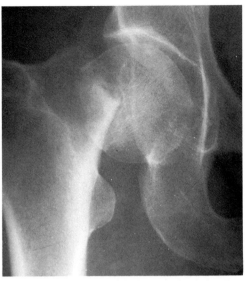

Fig. 6.3 Displaced subcapital fracture of the femur. *This fracture is often complicated by avascular necrosis.*

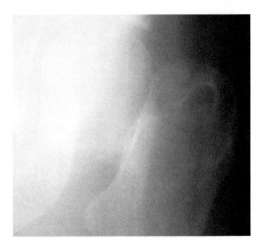

Fig. 6.4 Basicapital fracture. *The fracture extends through the medial cortex (calcar) of the femoral neck.*

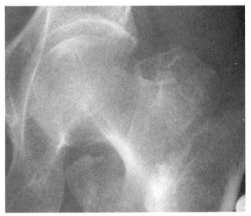

Fig. 6.5 Intertrochanteric fracture. *The fracture appears stable, with apposition of the fragments on the medial side. Note superior displacement of the lesser trochanter.*

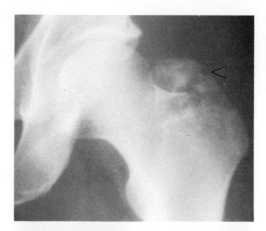

Fig. 6.6 Fracture of greater trochanter. *Note the transverse fracture* (arrow) *through the greater trochanter caused by avulsion of the hip abductors. Lesser trochanter avulsion is caused by the pull of the iliopsoas.*

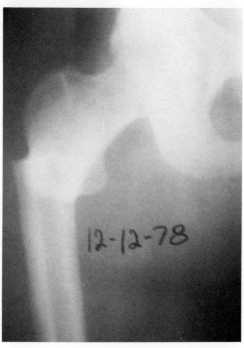

Fig. 6.7 Transverse subtrochanteric fracture. *Frontal projection shows a transverse fracture of the proximal femoral neck (subtrochanteric region) with superimposition of the fragments.*

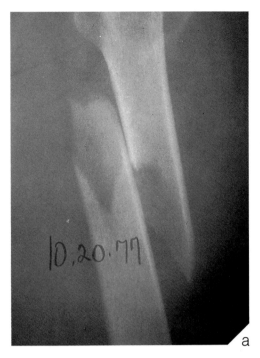
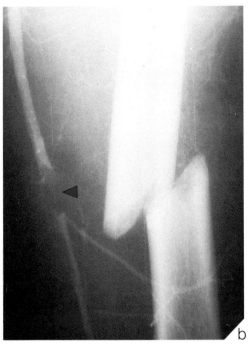

a

b

Fig. 6.8 Femoral shaft fractures. *a Oblique fracture of the femoral shaft. b Transverse* shaft fracture complicated by thrombosis of the superficial femoral artery (arrow).

Fig. 6.9 Femoral shaft fracture complicating hip joint prosthesis. *Note the transverse fracture at the tip of the prosthesis. This is the usual site of fracture in patients with metallic hip prostheses.*

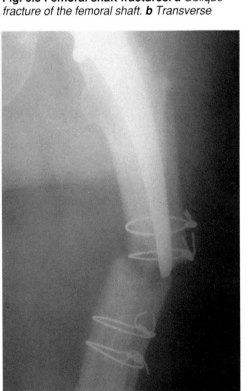

KNEE AND LEG FRACTURES

A wide variety of injuries occur in the vicinity of the knee joint. The distal femur may fracture either above the condyles (Fig. 6.10) or through them; these are known, respectively, as supracondylar and transcondylar fractures. Fractures of the individual condyles (condylar fractures) are less common (Fig. 6.11). Fractures of the tibial plateau are frequently depressed, and often are associated with ligamentous injuries. Avulsion fractures of the tibial spines, femoral epicondyles, fibular head, or anterior and posterior interspinous ridges are signs of a major injury to the supporting structures of the knee (Fig. 6.12). Disruption of the collateral ligaments can be confirmed by stress films (Fig. 6.13).

Patellar fractures, which are often caused by avulsion of the extensor mechanism, occur at the poles or in the body of the patella (Fig. 6.14). Internal fixation may be necessary if the fragments are displaced. Fractures of the upper pole must be differentiated from bipartite patella, a common developmental variant that is often bilateral: In bipartite patella, the defect is located in the upper outer quadrant and has sclerotic margins. Acute patellar dislocation is occasionally observed, but it is rare (Fig. 6.15).

Dislocations of the knee joint are usually caused by major deforming forces. They are relatively uncommon. Rotatory, posterior, medial, and lateral dislocations occur on occasion, but anterior dislocation is the variety most frequently seen (Fig. 6.16). An associated vascular injury, caused by stretching, is so common that arteriography is indicated even when there are no clinical signs of vascular compromise.

Tibial shaft fractures are among the most difficult fractures to manage and are associated with considerable morbidity. Because the anterior aspect of the tibia lies just beneath the subcutaneous tissues, shaft fractures are often open (and hence contaminated). Delayed union, nonunion, malunion, and osteomyelitis are not infrequent. In assessing such fractures, one must take into account five major variables: location, comminution, segmentation, displacement, and angulation (Figs. 6.17, 6.18). The fibular fracture that often accompanies tibial shaft fracture generally does not alter management. Fractures of the distal articular surface (plafond) and medial malleolus are more appropriately considered ankle fractures (see Ankle and Foot Fractures, below).

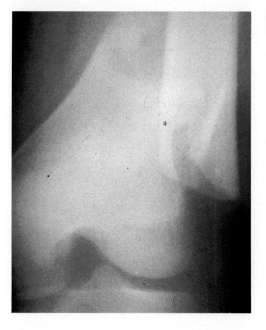

Fig. 6.10 Supracondylar femoral fracture.
Frontal projection shows an oblique supracondylar fracture with lateral displacement of the distal fragment.

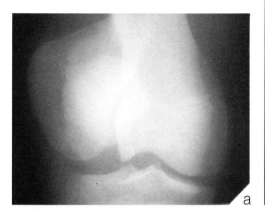
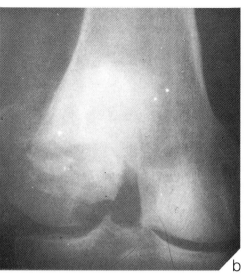

Fig. 6.11 Condylar fractures. *a* Frontal projection shows an isolated fracture of the lateral femoral condyle fracture that is angulated and displaced. *b* An isolated comminuted medial condyle fracture is seen in another patient.

Condylar fractures are much less common than intercondylar fractures; therefore, whenever a condylar fracture is identified, the films should be closely scrutinized for an intercondylar fracture line.

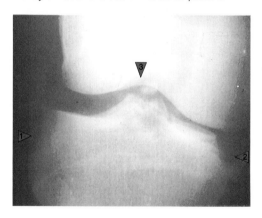

Fig. 6.12 Avulsion fractures. *Small avulsed fragments resulting from lateral collateral ligament avulsion (arrow 1), medial collateral ligament avulsion (arrow 2), and cruciate ligament avulsion (arrow 3), indicate that the integrity of those ligamentous structures is lost. The medial tibial plateau is fractured and slightly displaced.*

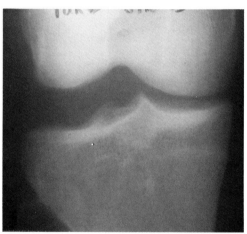

Fig. 6.13 Collateral ligament injury. *Varus stress film shows widening of the lateral knee compartment, which indicates that the lateral collateral ligament is unstable.*

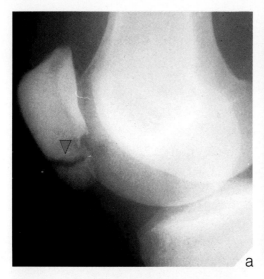

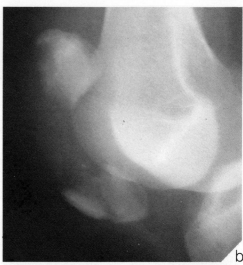

Fig. 6.14 Patellar fractures. *a Lateral projection shows a minimally displaced fracture of the inferior pole of the patella (arrow) caused by avulsion of the patellar ligament.* ***b*** *A com-* minuted and displaced fracture of the patella can be seen. These findings indicate that the surrounding retinaculum has been disrupted.

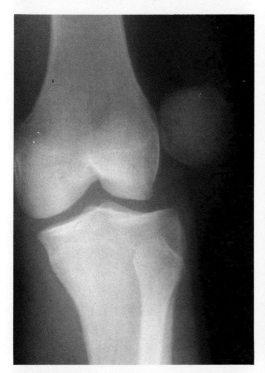

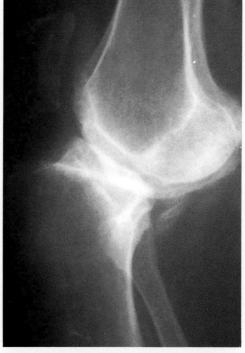

Fig. 6.15 Patellar dislocation. *Frontal projection shows a lateral dislocation of the patella. After treatment a CT scan should be performed to assess the extent of reduction and to search for occult fractures of the femoral condyles and patella.*

Fig. 6.16 Anterior dislocation of the knee. *Lateral projection shows marked anterior displacement of the tibia. This injury is frequently associated with damage to the popliteal artery; arteriography should be performed without hesitation if a vascular injury is suspected.*

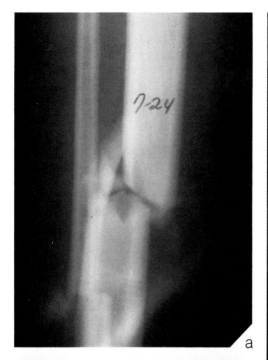

a

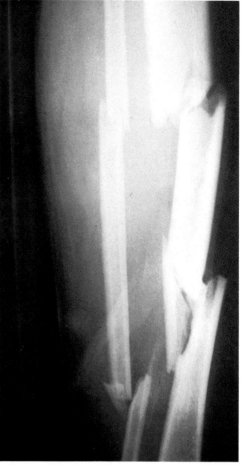

Fig. 6.18 Segmental fractures. *Frontal projection shows comminuted segmental fractures of the tibia. The shafts of both bones are broken into three segments. The tibial fragments protrude through the skin, making this an open injury. This type of fracture has a high incidence of infection and nonunion.*

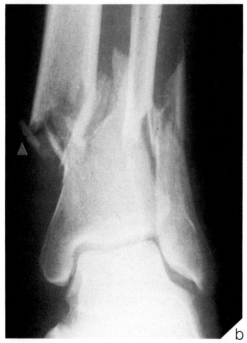

b

Fig. 6.17 Tibial shaft fractures. *a These mid-shaft tibial and fibular fractures were caused by direct impact by an automobile bumper. b In a skier, these fractures of the distal tibia and fibula result from varus, valgus, or anterior stress applied at the top of the ski boot; hence the term "boot-top fracture." A fracture fragment is protruding through the soft tissues (arrow).*

ANKLE AND FOOT FRACTURES

Ankle fractures can be highly complex injuries. To evaluate them properly, one must consider: the location and direction of fibular and malleolar fracture lines; the displacement of the fragments; the tilt of the talus; and the presence or absence of avulsions, foot fractures, and tibiofibular diastasis.

Among the more common types of ankle fracture are the following:

1. Adduction fracture (Fig. 6.19), which is often associated with collateral ligament disruption.
2. Supination-external rotation fracture (Figs. 6.20, 6.21), which may be associated with fracture of the distal fibula.
3. Pilon fracture (Fig. 6.22), which is associated with fragmentation of the distal tibia.
4. Osteochondral fracture of the talus (Fig. 6.23), which is often followed by avascular necrosis.
5. Pronation-external rotation fractures.

The foot is a complex of seven tarsal bones (the talus, the calcaneus, the navicular, the cuboid, and the medial, middle, and lateral cuneiforms), five metatarsals, and 14 phalanges (Fig. 6.24). Like the ankle, the foot can undergo various types of fractures. The calcaneus, for example, is subject to fracture at several points, including the insertion of the Achilles tendon (Fig. 6.25) and the vicinity of the subtalar joint (Fig. 6.26). Fractures of the midfoot and forefoot typically involve the metatarsals, the tarsometatarsal joint, the phalanges, or combinations thereof (Figs. 6.27–6.30).

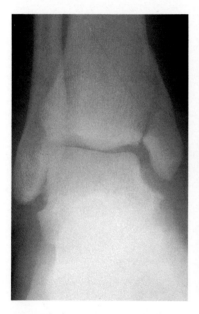

Fig. 6.19 Adduction fracture of the ankle. *The mechanism of injury can generally be reconstructed by analysis of the fracture lines. Since the fracture line follows an inferolateral-to-superomedial course through the medial malleolus, it can be presumed that the force was applied to the lateral aspect of the foot. In such injuries, the lateral collateral ligament may be disrupted as well.*

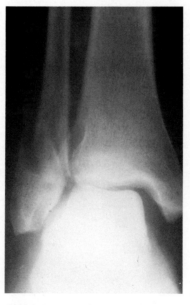

Fig. 6.20 Supination-external rotation fracture of the ankle. *The wide space between the medial malleolus and the talus indicates disruption of the deltoid ligament. In addition, there is an oblique fracture of the distal fibula.*

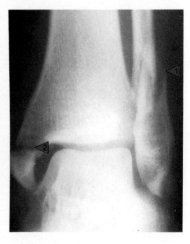

Fig. 6.21 Supination-external rotation fracture of the ankle. *In this patient there is a fracture of the medial malleolus (arrow 1) rather than a tear of the deltoid ligament. The spiral fracture of the distal fibular shaft (arrow 2) is characteristic of the mechanism of injury.*

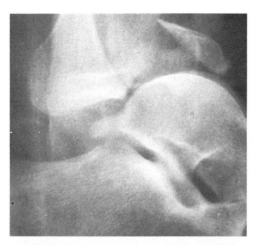

Fig. 6.22 Pilon fracture of the ankle. *Lateral projection shows fragmentation of the distal tibia. The mechanism of injury is axial compression of the ankle, which crushes the articular surface of the tibia against the dome of the talus.*

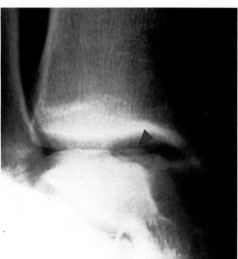

Fig. 6.23 Osteochondral fracture of the talus. *Oblique projection shows an osteochondral fracture (arrow) of the articular surface of the talus. Avascular necrosis is a frequent sequela of such injuries.*

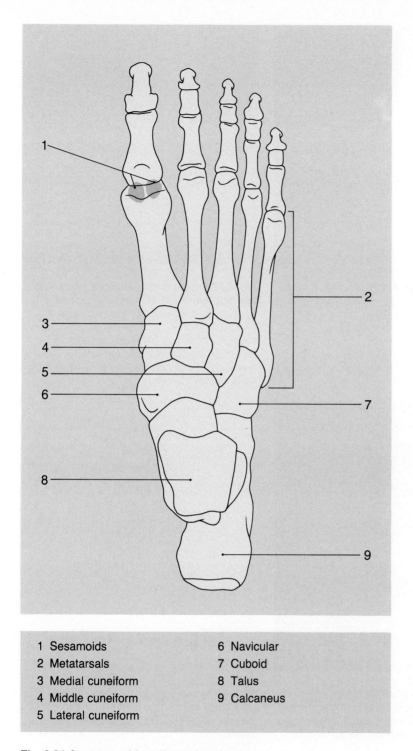

Fig. 6.24 Anatomy of foot (frontal projection).

1 Sesamoids   6 Navicular
2 Metatarsals   7 Cuboid
3 Medial cuneiform   8 Talus
4 Middle cuneiform   9 Calcaneus
5 Lateral cuneiform

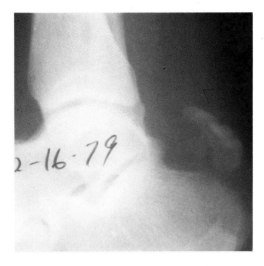

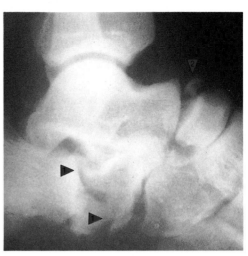

Fig. 6.25 Avulsion of Achilles' tendon insertion. *Lateral projection shows a bone fragment (arrow) that has been avulsed from the posterosuperior margin of the calcaneus.*

Fig. 6.26 Fracture of calcaneus extending into subtalar joint. *A man jumped from a third-story window and landed on his heel. Lateral projection shows a comminuted depressed fracture of the calcaneus with disruption of the subtalar joint (arrows 1). There is also a small avulsion fracture of the tarsal navicular (arrow 2).*

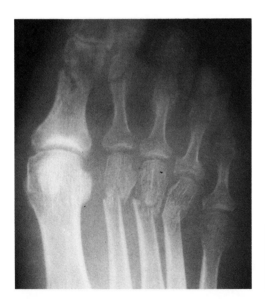

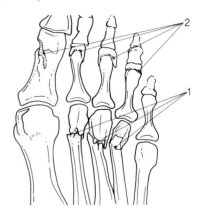

1 Fracture of metatarsal neck	2 Fracture of proximal phalangeal shaft

Fig. 6.27 Fractures of metatarsals and proximal phalanges. *While crossing the street this man was hit by a car which apparently ran over his foot. Frontal projection of the foot shows fractures of the second, third, and fourth metatarsal necks, and fractures of the first, second, third, and fourth proximal phalangeal shafts.*

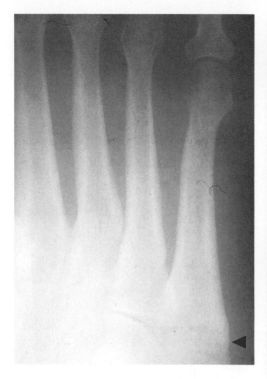

Fig. 6.28 Jones Fracture. *Oblique projection of the foot shows an avulsion of the peroneus brevis tendon from the styloid process of the fifth metatarsal (arrow).*

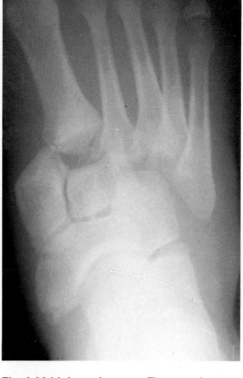

Fig. 6.29 Lisfranc fracture. *There are fractures of the bases of the second, third, and fourth metatarsals, as well as dislocations of the tarsometatarsal joints. These injuries are usually caused by violent deforming forces that disrupt the supporting ligaments of the tarso-metatarsal joints and result in dislocations. Chronic pain and discomfort are common sequelae of this injury.*

Fig. 6.30 March fracture. *Note exuberant callus (arrow) along second metatarsal shaft, a typical site for stress fractures in joggers and military recruits.*

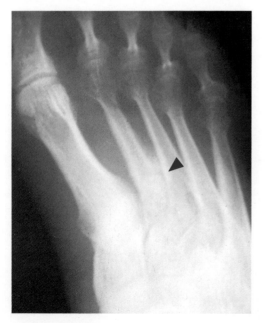

SECTION II:

Radiology of Nonskeletal Trauma

CHAPTER SEVEN

*H*ead and Neck

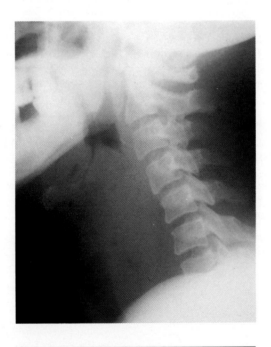

Until recently, the application of radiology to the evaluation of acute soft-tissue injuries of the head and neck was limited to plain radiographs and angiography. Computed tomography (CT) has dramatically altered the role of imaging in the evaluation and treatment of injuries of the head and neck and is now the diagnostic procedure of choice in the assessment of head trauma. Magnetic resonance imaging (MRI) shows great promise and indeed may prove to be even more sensitive than CT in detecting and ascertaining the prognosis of brain injuries.

Pneumocephalus (air within the head) is usually caused by a fracture of the base of the skull or the frontal sinus. It may present as an air–fluid level or as mottled air within the sulci of the brain (Fig. 7.1).

CT is very useful in the evaluation of injuries of the face and neck. The excellent density discrimination of CT allows visualization of the orbital contents. Injuries of the globe and the extent of intraorbital hemorrhage, as well as herniation and entrapment of extraocular muscles associated with fractures of the orbital floor, are clearly seen (Figs. 7.2, 7.3). Foreign bodies (e.g., bullet fragments) can be precisely localized (Fig. 7.4). Fractures and dislocations of the laryngeal cartilages also can be demonstrated (Fig. 7.5).

PENETRATING NECK WOUNDS

Radiology plays a critical role in the assessment of penetrating neck wounds; a thorough radiologic evaluation can sometimes obviate surgical exploration. Imaging studies used to evaluate penetrating neck wounds include plain films of the neck, esophagography, arteriography, sialography, CT,

and fluoroscopy. The choice of imaging technique depends upon the site of penetration.

Hemorrhage, subcutaneous emphysema (SQE), and injuries of the epiglottis and cervical airway are readily demonstrated on plain films. A retropharyngeal hematoma is identified on the lateral projection by noting an increase in the soft tissue between the anterior aspect of the vertebral body and the airway (Figs. 7.6, 7.7). Injuries of the larynx and traumatic vocal cord paralysis can be diagnosed by careful scrutiny of the plain films (Figs. 7.8, 7.9). Sialography may be needed to show disruption of the salivary ducts (Fig. 7.10).

SQE may be innocuous (i.e., air introduced mechanically when the skin was penetrated) or it can indicate a pharyngeal or esophageal perforation (Fig. 7.11). Barium swallow should be done in patients with SQE to exclude or confirm pharyngoesophageal injury (Figs. 7.12–7.14). Hypertonic, water-soluble contrast media (e.g., Gastrografin) can cause pulmonary edema if aspirated and should not be used for this purpose.

It is useful to classify penetrating neck wounds according to the site of penetration (Fig. 7.15). Zone I injuries occur in the vicinity of the thoracic inlet. Zone II injuries occur in the midneck. Zone III injuries involve the high neck, near the base of the skull. Injuries of the posterior triangle of the neck are considered separately. Arteriography is often needed to evaluate penetrating injuries, especially those in Zones I and III, which may be associated with an occult vascular injury. Thromboses, pseudoaneurysms, and arteriovenous fistulas are the most common abnormalities demonstrated by angiography (Figs. 7.16–7.19).

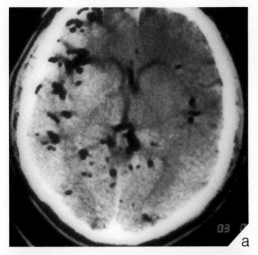

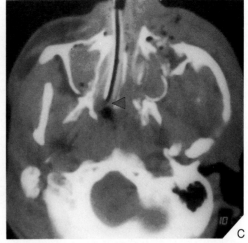

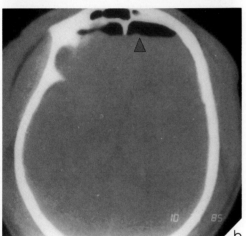

Fig. 7.1 Pneumocephalus. *a This patient sustained a basal skull fracture. CT shows air within the sulci.* ***b*** *CT in a patient with a complex facial fracture shows pneumocephalus (arrow), with gas–fluid levels overlying the frontal cortex* ***c***. *A more caudal cut shows a nasogastric tube (arrow) passing through a fracture in the floor of the anterior cranial fossa into the cranial cavity. Oroesophageal intubation should be performed in patients with complex maxillofacial injuries to avoid this complication.*

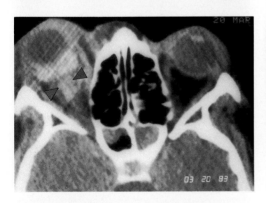

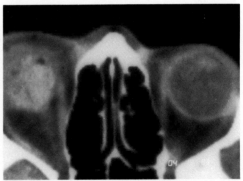

Fig. 7.2 Intraconal hematoma. *Axial CT shows a high-attenuation mass representing a hematoma (arrows) behind the right globe, within the cone of the extraocular muscles. Retrobulbar hematomas, which are located within a closed compartment that contains the optic nerve, may result in optic nerve infarction and blindness.*

Fig. 7.3 Ruptured globe. *The right globe is filled with blood and air and none of the normal anatomic features can be identified (compare with a normal left globe).*

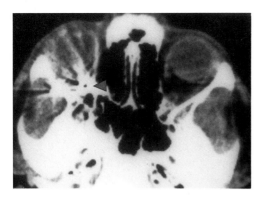

Fig. 7.4 Intraorbital foreign body. *In this patient, traumatic blindness was caused by a gunshot wound. The bullet fragment (arrow) occupies the location of the optic nerve.*

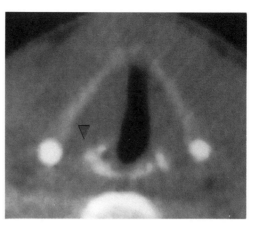

Fig. 7.5 Laryngeal fracture. *Axial CT scan shows swelling of the right vocal cord and subluxation of the right cricoarytenoid joint (arrow).*

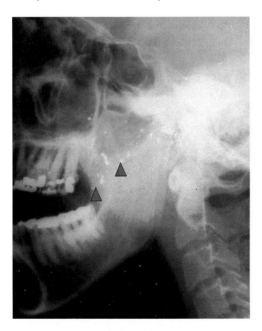

Fig. 7.6 Nasopharyngeal hematoma. *A lateral film shows a large soft-tissue mass that displaces the nasopharyngeal and oropharyngeal air column anteriorly. Note the bullet fragments overlying the body of C1 (arrows). Arteriography (not shown) demonstrated a laceration of the internal carotid artery.*

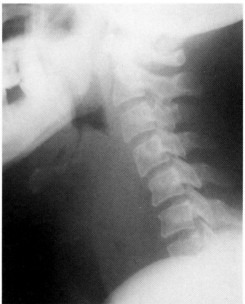

Fig. 7.7 Hypopharyngeal hematoma. *A lateral film shows anterior displacement of the hypopharyngeal air column and widening of the prevertebral space. The prevertebral space, measured between the anterior aspect of C4 and the posterior aspect of the airway should be no greater than 40 percent of the anteroposterior diameter of C4.*

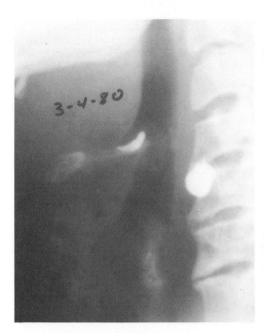

Fig. 7.8 Epiglottic hematoma. *A lateral film shows swelling of the epiglottis, causing partial obstruction of the airway. Note the bullet fragment in the epiglottis.*

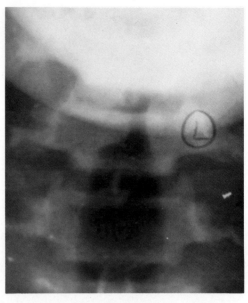

Fig. 7.9 Vocal cord paralysis. *A frontal soft-tissue radiograph, obtained during quiet breathing, in a patient with a gunshot wound of the neck shows lack of abduction of the right vocal cord. Traumatic vocal cord paralysis may be caused by a high vagal or recurrent laryngeal nerve injury. An associated injury of the carotid artery should be suspected in a patient with vagal nerve trauma due to a penetrating injury.*

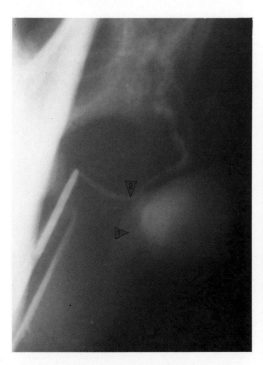

Fig. 7.10 Salivary duct laceration. *A carotid sialogram (obtained after cannulation of Stensen's duct) in a patient with a penetrating wound of the cheek shows extravasation of contrast material* (arrow 1) *from the partially lacerated duct* (arrow 2).

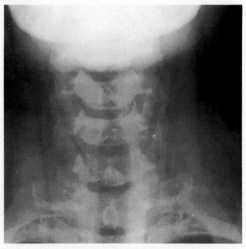

Fig. 7.11 Subcutaneous emphysema. *Air outlines all of the fascial planes of the neck. This appearance may be caused by air dissecting from the mediastinum or lung, from the trachea or larynx, from the hypopharynx, or from the penetrating wound itself.*

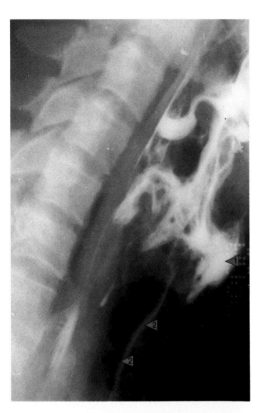

Fig. 7.12 Hypopharyngeal perforation.
Lateral film of esophagram shows subcutaneous emphysema and extravasation of barium (arrow 1) *from the hypopharynx. Note the contrast material outlining the anterior wall of the trachea* (arrows 2). *This could be caused by aspiration or by a tracheopharyngeal fistula.*

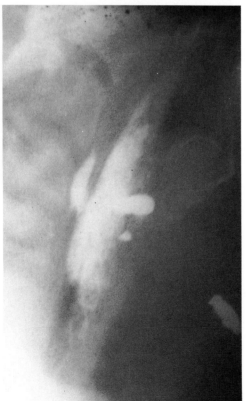

Fig. 7.13 Laceration of the cervical esophagus. *The barium column is irregular and is not confined within the sharply delineated outline of the esophagus.*

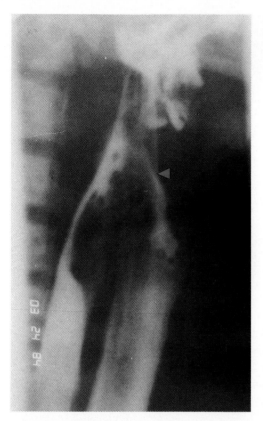

Fig. 7.14 Traumatic tracheoesophageal fistula. *Lateral film of esophagram shows tears of both the anterior wall of the pharyngoesophageal junction and the posterior wall of the trachea* (arrow). *Note the massive extravasation of barium into the trachea.*

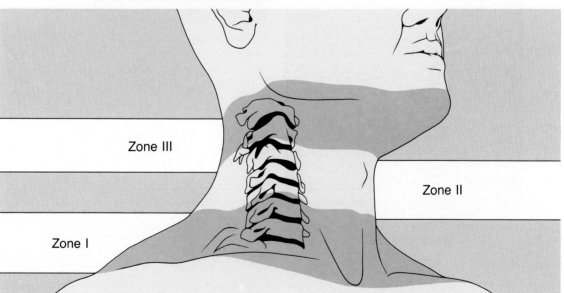

Fig. 7.15 Zones of the neck. *Penetrating anterior neck injuries are classified according to the location of* *the entry wound (Zone I, II, or III injuries). Occult arterial injuries are associated with Zone I and III injuries.*

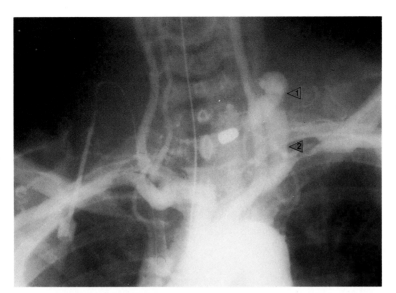

Fig. 7.16 Zone I arterial injury.
Aortography is the initial study of choice for penetrating wounds in this zone. This patient has an arteriovenous fistula between the vertebral artery and the jugular vein. A pseudoaneurysm of the vertebral artery (arrow 1) and early filling of the jugular vein (arrow 2) can be appreciated on a film obtained during the early arterial phase.

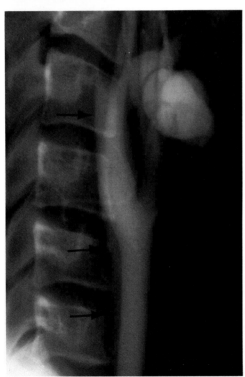

Fig. 7.17 Zone II arterial injury. *Selective carotid and, when indicated, vertebral catheterization are necessary to characterize injuries in this zone. This study shows extravasation from the external carotid artery and early opacification of the internal jugular vein (arrows).*

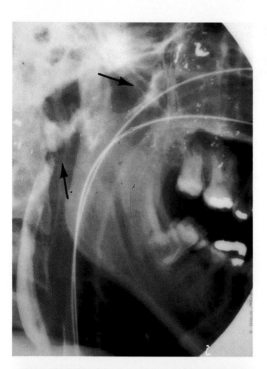

Fig. 7.18 Zone III arterial injury. *Injuries in this zone are often clinically subtle. In this patient, selective internal carotid arteriography of the internal carotid artery shows contrast extravasation* (arrows) *from the carotid artery into the pharynx.*

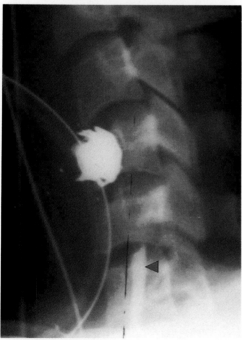

Fig. 7.19 Posterior triangle arterial injury. *A selective arteriogram shows occlusion of the vertebral artery* (arrow).

CHAPTER EIGHT

Chest

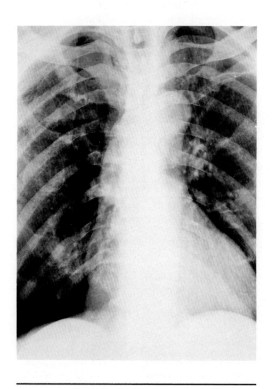

The initial radiographic examination of the multiply injured patient should include a frontal radiograph of the chest. This inexpensive, quickly performed study can detect high-risk—even life-threatening—injuries. The initial chest film is a screening study and is performed with the patient supine. Once the patient has been resuscitated and assessed, an upright chest film can be obtained if necessary.

Analysis of the initial chest film should be directed first at determining whether it is of adequate quality. Attempting to read a film that is "unreadable" due to motion, poor radiographic technique, or other artifacts can lead to serious errors in interpretation and management. Following a simple checklist will minimize the likelihood of error. Compare the lucency (transradiancy) of each hemithorax. Increased or decreased transradiancy of one or both hemithoraces can be due to abnormalities of the chest wall, pleural spaces, or lungs. Define the soft-tissue structures (heart, aorta, vascular markings, and diaphragm). Are they sharp? Are they obscured by lung or pleural opacities? Check the location of the trachea, pulmonary hila, diaphragm, and heart. Assess the size, shape, and position of the medi-astinum. Is all the "hardware" where it belongs? (Fig. 8.1).

PNEUMOTHORAX

Decreased opacity usually indicates pneumothorax, mastectomy, or increased opacity of the contralateral thorax. When there is a moderate amount of air in the pleural space, the vascular markings do not extend to the chest wall; the visceral pleura can be identified as a sharp linear density demarcated by air in the pleural cavity and air in the lung (Figs. 8.2, 8.3). Displacement of the lung away from the chest wall is usually most conspicuous in the apical and lateral regions. In a tension pneumothorax, the mediastinum is displaced to the opposite side and the diaphragm is de-pressed downward (Fig. 8.4). A small or moderate-size pneumothorax may appear as a lucent band between the mediastinum and the medial edge of the lung. In some instances, intrapleural air may be difficult to detect on a supine film. Clues to the diagnosis include an unusual lucency of the epigastric region, deepening of the ipsilateral costophrenic sulcus, or a sharply outlined apical fat pad.

CT is a more sensitive means of identifying intrapleural air than plain chest radiographs, espe-

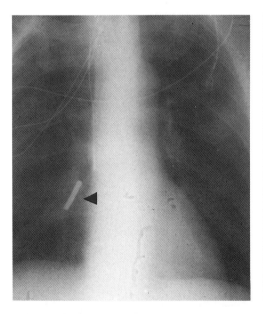

Fig. 8.1 Misplaced feeding tube. *In this multiply injured patient, the tip of a feeding tube* (arrow) *can be seen in the right lower lobe bronchus. It was inadvertently introduced into the trachea during resuscitation.*

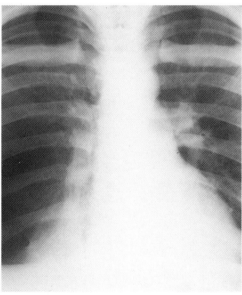

Fig. 8.2 Complete pneumothorax. *The right hemithorax is hyperlucent. The right lower lobe is collapsed. No lung markings are seen in the lower chest.*

cially in acutely injured patients who cannot be moved from the recumbent position. However, a pneumothorax can be missed on CT unless wide window settings are used. Since the patient is supine, intrapleural air collects superior to the lung and is visualized as a lucent stripe beneath the anterior chest wall (Fig. 8.5).

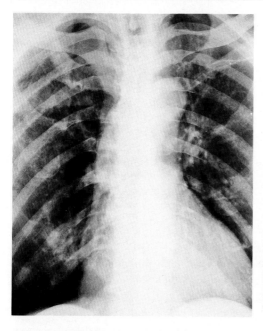

Fig. 8.3 Moderate pneumothorax (hemo-pneumothorax). *The linear opacity represents the visceral pleura outlined by air within the lung and in the pleural space.*

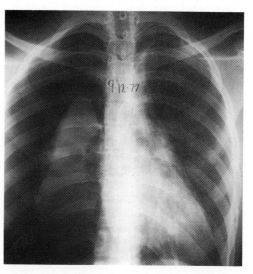

Fig. 8.4 Tension pneumothorax. *The right hemithorax is hyperlucent. Increased intrapleural pressure is manifested by contralateral displacement of the mediastinum and depression of the ipsilateral diaphragm.*

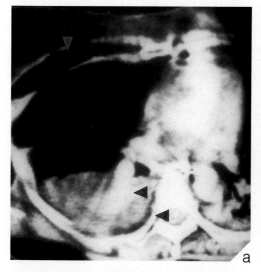

a

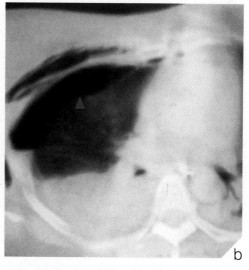

b

Fig. 8.5 Hemopneumothorax shown by CT. *a CT of the right chest, photographed at a narrow window setting, shows air beneath the pectoral muscles (arrow 1), blood in the pleural space (arrow 2), and consolidated lung (arrow 3). A pneumothorax is not seen. b The same slice photographed at a "lung" window shows air in the pleural space (arrow).*

PLEURAL AND PARENCHYMAL ABNORMALITIES

In the acutely injured patient, increased opacity of a hemithorax can result from: Blood; fluid; or secretions within the pleura (hydrothorax or hemothorax), the lung (lung contusion, hematoma, collapse, aspiration, or pulmonary edema), or in the chest wall. On a supine film, a hemothorax appears as hazy opacity through which, on a properly exposed radiograph, the vascular markings may be seen. A large amount of fluid will displace the mediastinum into the contralateral hemithorax (Fig. 8.6). A supine film may fail to demonstrate a small amount of pleural fluid; conversely, pleural fluid may be suggested when none is present. A lateral decubitus film with the abnormal side down can be obtained to confirm the presence of pleural fluid if the patient's condition permits.

A number of disease processes (e.g., contusion, aspiration, edema, pneumonia, and atelectasis) result in air space abnormalities. Chest films or CT show fluffy, ill-defined opacities that obscure the pulmonary vascular markings and air bronchograms (tubular radiolucencies surrounded by opacity) (Fig. 8.7). *Lung contusions* are nonlobar in distribution, often paralleling a rib, and typically resolve rapidly within 2 to 3 days unless complicated by pneumonia (Fig. 8.8). If there is an associated *lung hematoma*, an oval or round mass will become apparent as the contusion clears. Lung hematomas resolve slowly (weeks to months) and may cavitate (Fig. 8.9). *Atelectasis* is a common cause of air space abnormality in the injured patient. It is usually lobar or segmental and results in a shift of the mediastinum into the ipsilateral hemithorax and/or elevation of the ipsilateral diaphragm (Fig. 8.10). *Aspiration* is a common cause of parenchymal disease in injured patients, especially drug abusers and those with head trauma. The chest film characteristically shows opacification of air spaces in areas associated with posteriorly directed bronchi.

A well-demarcated parenchymal lucency can represent a traumatic pneumatocele (Fig. 8.11), cavitating hematoma (see Fig. 8.9b), lung abscess, or a thoracostomy tube tract (Fig. 8.12). Correlation with the clinical findings will suggest the correct diagnosis.

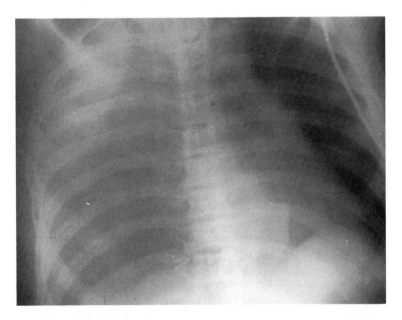

Fig. 8.6 Massive hemothorax. *A supine chest film of a patient who had sustained a gunshot wound shows opacification of the right hemithorax with a contralateral mediastinal shift. Vascular markings can be identified in the right lower lung field. Thoracentesis yielded 3 liters of blood.*

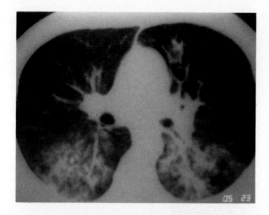

Fig. 8.7 Air space disease shown by CT.
Fluffy opacities that obscure the pulmonary vessels, producing air bronchograms, are characteristic of air space disease. Likely causes in a patient with a chest injury include contusion, aspiration, collapse, and hemorrhage.

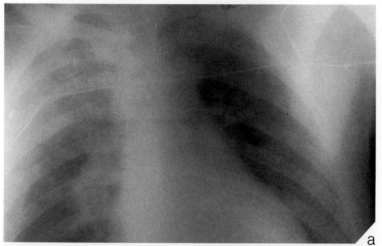

a

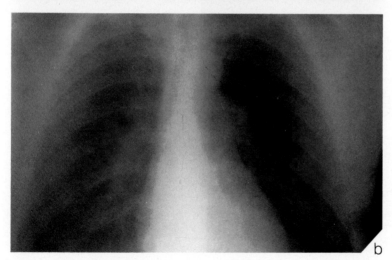

b

Fig. 8.8 Lung contusion. *a The chest film shows increased opacity in the right upper lung zone. The pulmonary vascularity is obscured. Note that the distribution is nonlobar in nature, conforming to the area of the fractured ribs. **b** A follow-up film on the following day shows resolutions of the opacity, confirming the diagnosis of contusion.*

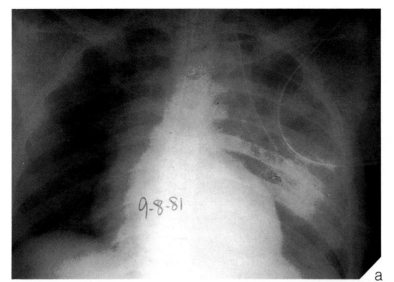

Fig. 8.9 Pulmonary contusion and hematoma. *a* A large parenchymal opacity consisting of a central oval density and fluffy peripheral opacities is seen in the left lower lobe. *b* Ten days later, the fluffy peripheral opacities (contusion) have cleared, while the central density (hematoma) has cavitated. The radiographic appearance of a cavitary hematoma is indistinguishable from that of a lung abscess or pneumatocele; differentiation is based on clinical criteria.

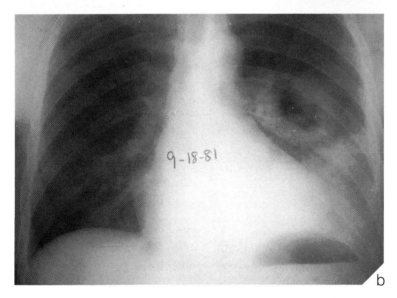

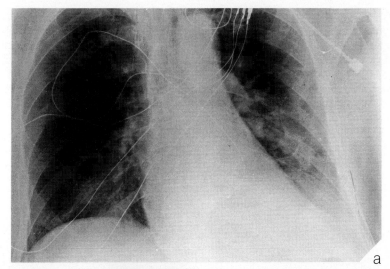

a

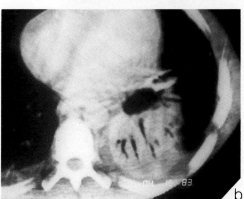

b

Fig. 8.10 Atelectasis. *a* Chest film shows collapse of the left lower lobe with an ipsilateral shift of the heart and mediastinum. The left diaphragm is not visible because the lower left lobe is airless. *b* CT shows a consolidation of the left lower lobe. The crowded, air-filled bronchi are outlined against the surrounding opacified lung.

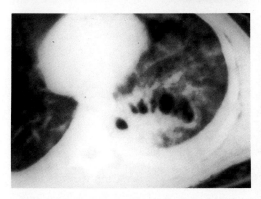

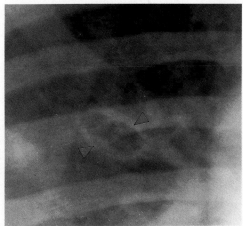

Fig. 8.11 Traumatic pneumatocele. *This patient's chest was compressed against the steering wheel in a head-on collision with another vehicle. CT performed soon after admission shows a cavity with surrounding air space opacity. A traumatic pneumatocele that results from alveolar rupture caused by increased intrathoracic pressure cannot be distinguished radiographically from an abscess; in this case, the clinical history and early appearance of the parenchymal lucency suggested the correct diagnosis.*

Fig. 8.12 Chest tube tract. *The small oval radiolucency (arrows), which might be mistaken for a pneumatocele or a lung abscess, represents air within the tract of a recently removed thoracostomy tube.*

AORTIC INJURIES

A careful analysis of the mediastinum is a mandatory part of the radiologic evaluation of any patient with a major blunt chest injury. Widening of the mediastinum (greater than 8 cm on an upright or supine film) is considered presumptive evidence of mediastinal bleeding; in this context, the possibility of an aortic laceration must be seriously considered (Fig. 8.13). If possible, an upright 6-foot chest film should be obtained to exclude artefactual mediastinal widening; however, it is *never* safe to assume that a widened mediastinum is caused by radiographic projection. Other plain-film findings suggesting aortic injury include loss of definition of the descending aorta or the aortic knob, rightward displacement of a nasogastric tube or the trachea, and depression of the left mainstem bronchus. If possible, these findings should be confirmed with a well-positioned upright film.

Aortography should be performed whenever clinical and/or radiographic findings suggest a mediastinal hematoma. Aortographic manifestations of traumatic aortic laceration include the presence of an intimal flap (Fig. 8.14), saccular extravasation, and pseudoaneurysm formation (Fig. 8.15a). With rare exceptions, the aortic lesion occurs just beyond the origin of the left subclavian artery.

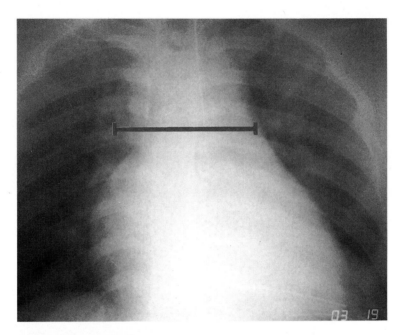

Fig. 8.13 Hemomediastinum. *The superior mediastinum is widened, measuring greater than 8 cm (bar). The aorta is not visualized on this supine film. In a patient with these findings, the next step would be to repeat the chest film with a target-film distance of 72 in. and the patient upright. If an upright film cannot be obtained (or if it confirms the mediastinal widening), aortography must be done to exclude an aortic injury.*

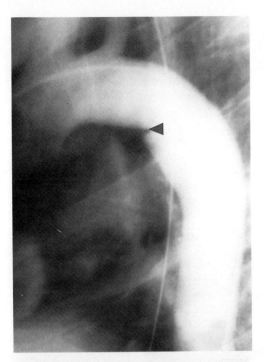

Fig. 8.14 Aortic intimal flap. *A lateral aortogram shows a small, subtle linear radiolucency (arrow) that represents an elevated intimal flap at the site of an aortic laceration. Note that the descending aorta is wider than the more proximal aortic arch due to the presence of contrast material in the wall of the descending aorta, indicating intramural dissection.*

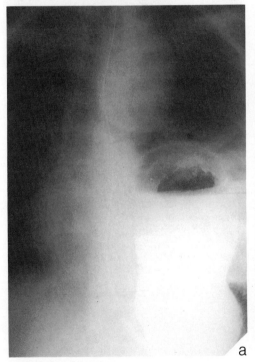

a

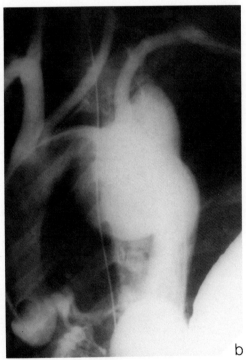

b

Fig. 8.15 Aortic pseudoaneurysm and traumatic diaphragmatic hernia. *Four years earlier, this man fractured his femur in a car accident. A chest injury was not diagnosed during that hospitalization. **a** Erect film of the upper gastrointestinal area shows enlargement of the aortic arch, displacement of the trachea to the right, and downward displacement of the left mainstem bronchus. The stomach has herniated into the left chest through an anterior defect in the diaphragm. **b** Right posterior oblique projection of aortogram shows a large saccular pseudoaneurysm arising just beyond the origin of the left subclavian artery.*

INJURIES OF THE DIAPHRAGM

Diaphragmatic injuries may be very subtle. Rapid accumulation of pleural fluid after a diagnostic abdominal peritoneal lavage indicates a diaphragmatic tear, while elevation of the diaphragm is a suggestive finding. Abdominal viscera (stomach, colon, liver, and bowel) may herniate through the defect into the thoracic cavity (Fig. 8.15b). Depending on the circumstances, barium studies, liver–spleen scintigraphy, CT, or angiography can be used to confirm the diagnosis (Figs. 8.16–8.18).

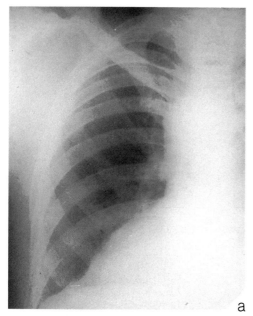

a

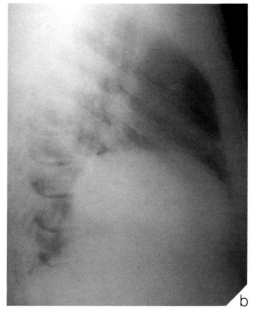

b

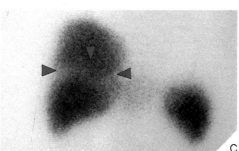

c

Fig. 8.16 Right diaphragmatic laceration with hepatic herniation. *This man sustained a closed chest injury in a fall 5 years before. **a** Frontal and **b** lateral chest radiographs show apparent elevation of the right hemidiaphragm. **c** A TC[99m] sulfur colloid liver–spleen scan shows a photon-deficient band (arrows) at the level of the diaphragm, indicating displacement of the liver into the right hemithorax. At operation there was a large anterior defect in the diaphragm with upward herniation of the right lobe of the liver.*

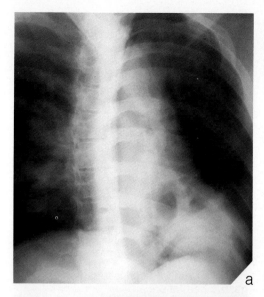

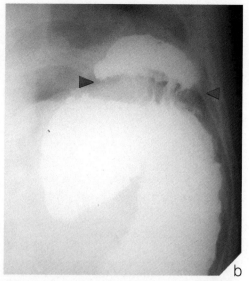

Fig. 8.17 Diaphragmatic laceration with colonic herniation. *a* *A frontal chest radiograph shows a density containing multiple radiolucencies at the base of the left hemithorax. This appearance is consistent with a lung abscess, empyema and/or upward herniation of abdominal contents. **b** Barium enema shows an "hourglass" deformity (arrows) of the barium column. Operation revealed herniation of the colon through a small hole in the left diaphragm. **c** Chest film of another patient with herniation of the colon through a traumatic diaphragmatic hernia shows lucencies at the left base (arrow 1) that represent a strangulated bowel. The oval opacity along the lateral chest wall (arrow 2) represents an empyema secondary to colonic perforation.*

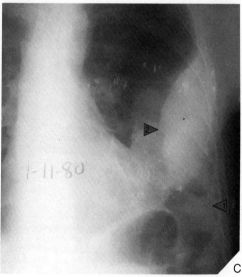

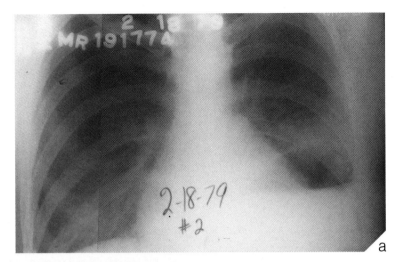

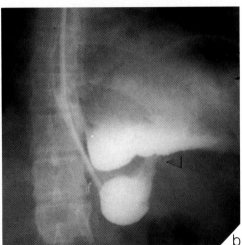

Fig. 8.18 Diaphragmatic laceration with gastric herniation. *a* Chest film shows upward displacement of the gastric shadow. *b* An upper GI series confirms herniation of the stomach into the left hemithorax. Note the annular constriction of the stomach (arrow) *at the site of the diaphragmatic defect.*

C H A P T E R   N I N E

*A*bdomen and
Gastrointestinal Tract

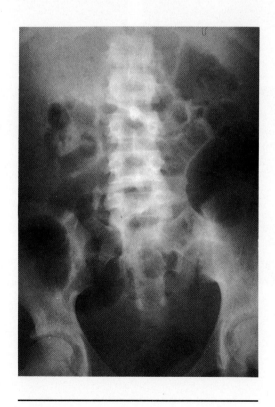

The radiological evaluation of abdominal trauma usually begins with plain films. While plain radiography has limited applicability in this era of sophisticated imaging techniques, it remains most useful in localizing intraabdominal bullets and opaque foreign bodies (Figs. 9.1, 9.2), and in detecting free air. Enlargement of the spleen is a classic, though uncommon, plain film manifestation of an intracapsular hematoma (Fig. 9.3).

More sophisticated imaging techniques include scintigraphy, ultrasonography, angiography, and CT. At our trauma center, we rely heavily on CT—the only imaging modality that can simultaneously evaluate all of the abdominal organs—as the primary imaging modality, especially for blunt trauma. Angiography is used to evaluate patients with continuing blood loss, some of whom may be candidates for percutaneous embolization techniques.

CT: TECHNICAL CONSIDERATIONS

Careful patient preparation is essential if CT is to be reliable in the evaluation of intraabdominal pathology. It is our practice to administer a 1- to 3-percent solution of water-soluble contrast orally or by nasogastric tube (in 300 ml aliquots: 60 min, 15 min, and immediately before scanning), in order to opacify the gastrointestinal tract.

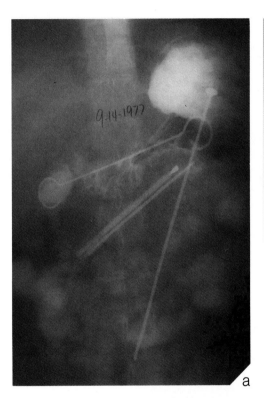

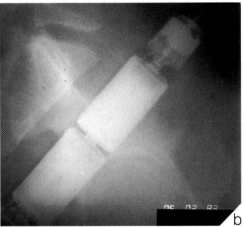

Fig. 9.1 Foreign bodies in the gastrointestinal tract. *a This psychotic person swallowed multiple foreign bodies, including a fork, a spoon handle, wires, and pens. **b** A vibrator lodged in the rectum.*

Intravenous enhancement is necessary to distinguish clearly intraparenchymal hematomas from the surrounding parenchyma. We administer a bolus of 150 ml of a 60-percent urographic agent concentration of radiopaque contrast. Artifacts, particularly those due to metallic objects, can seriously degrade the images. Before scanning, the nasogastric should be withdrawn into the esophagus and ECG leads removed from the area to be scanned. The examination should include the entire abdomen and pelvis. Since intraperitoneal blood tends to accumulate in the pelvis, this region should be carefully studied.

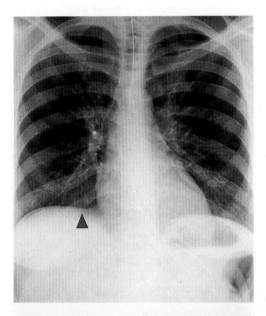

Fig. 9.2 Free intraabdominal air.
Pneumoperitoneum is best seen in the upright position of the chest and abdomen (arrow).

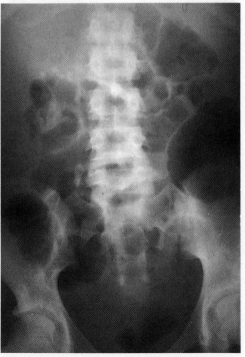

Fig. 9.3 Subcapsular hematoma of the spleen. *Plain film of the abdomen shows displacement of colonic gas from the flanks by intraperitoneal fluid (hemorrhage). The soft tissue mass in the left upper quadrant represents an enlarged spleen.*

HEMOPERITONEUM AND HEMATOMAS

CT is a very sensitive method for detecting and determining the extent of hemoperitoneum, which is imaged as a fluid of high or mixed attenuation. Intraperitoneal blood preferentially collects in the pelvis, in the subphrenic spaces, in the paracolic gutters, and in Morison's pouch (Fig. 9.4).

The appearance of contained hematomas varies with the age of the hematoma, the technique of contrast enhancement, and the photographic display parameters used. Very high attenuation (density) suggests active arterial bleeding, especially if the contrast material has been properly administered. Acutely clotted blood is isodense with circulating blood. Within 2 hours of clotting, the density of clotted blood is greater than that of flowing blood. Over a period of weeks, hematomas becomes heterogeneous and hypodense regions appear. Layering of sediment within the hematoma is quite common. Chronic hematomas are usually of water density and may have a thick, fibrotic rim.

Periparenchymal hematomas often obscure the margins of an organ, which, under normal circumstances, are sharply delineated. Intraparenchymal hematomas are contained within the affected organ. Lacerations appear as cracks and fissures within an organ.

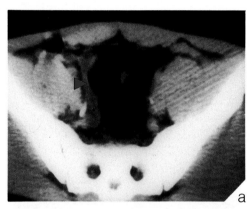

a

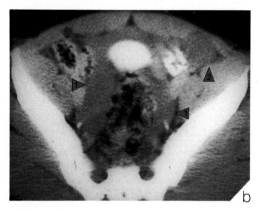

b

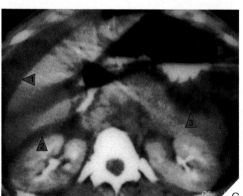

c

Fig. 9.4 Hemoperitoneum. *CT findings in three patients are shown.* ***a*** *An enhanced CT scan shows a small amount of intraperitoneal blood (arrow) in the pelvis adjacent to the sigmoid colon.* ***b*** *In a second patient, an enhanced CT scan shows a larger amount of free blood (arrows 1) in the pelvis. Fluid (arrow 2) is also seen adjacent to the descending colon.* ***c*** *An enhanced CT scan shows a massive hemoperitoneum in a third patient. Blood is present in both subphrenic spaces (arrow 1), Morrison's pouch (arrow 2), and the lesser sac (arrow 3).*

INJURIES OF SOLID VISCERA

CT is very accurate in identifying fractures and hematomas within the liver (Figs. 9.5, 9.6), as well as bile lakes ("bilomas") due to laceration of bile ducts (Fig. 9.7). Selective arteriography may demonstrate an active bleeding site or pseudoaneurysm (Figs. 9.8–9.11). While radionuclide scans can demonstrate subcapsular and intraparenchymal hematomas (Fig. 9.12), their main role is in the evaluation of traumatic bile leaks (Fig. 9.13).

Splenic hematomas (Figs. 9.14–9.17) and lacerations (Fig. 9.18) are clearly depicted by CT. Nuclear scintigraphy will also demonstrate acute splenic injuries, though it is less informative than CT (Fig. 9.19). Angiography is performed in stable patients to determine whether active bleeding is present and whether percutaneous embolization is feasible (Fig. 9.20).

Pancreatic injuries are often subtle on CT; loss of definition of the pancreatic contour and swelling of the gland are common but nonspecific findings. A pancreatic hematoma may be imaged as a low-attenuation region within the gland (Fig. 9.21). A pseudocyst may develop weeks or months after the acute injury (Fig. 9.22). Angiography may show extravasation from pancreatic vessels, especially in penetrating injuries (Fig. 9.23).

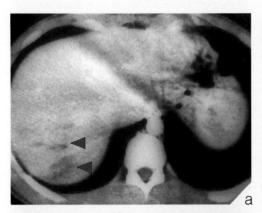

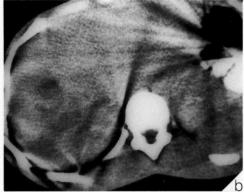

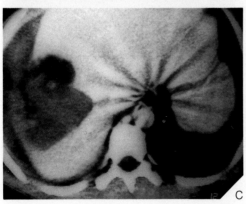

Fig. 9.5 Hepatic hematomas. *CT findings in three patients with blunt abdominal injuries are shown.* **a** *An enhanced scan shows a small, contained intrahepatic laceration. Several linear, low-attenuation areas* (arrows) *can be identified in the posterior aspect of the right hepatic lobe. There is no evidence of hemoperitonuem.* **b** *An enhanced CT scan shows a moderate-size hepatic hematoma, which appears as an area of diminished attenuation within the right lobe of the liver.* **c** *A large, mixed-attenuation hematoma is seen in the right lobe of the liver on this contrast-enhanced scan. Note the hemorrhage surrounding the hematoma, which is not contained by Glisson's capsule.*

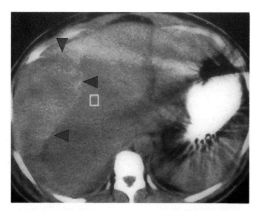

Fig. 9.6 Subcapsular hematoma of the liver.
The high-attenuation area (arrows) on the lateral aspect of the right hepatic lobe in this unenhanced CT scan. represents a subcapsular hematoma. The liver parenchyma, which is less dense than the hematoma, has a concave outer border. (The cursor is over the liver.) If intravenous contrast material has been given, the density (attenuation) of the liver parenchyma would have increased and the hematoma would have appeared less dense *than the liver.*

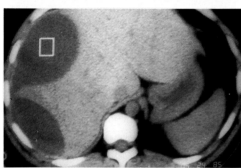

Fig. 9.7 Subcapsular "biloma." *The bilobed low-attenuation area along the lateral aspect of the right hepatic lobe seen on this unenhanced scan represents a subcapsular collection of bile secondary to a liver laceration. Percutaneous aspiration will differentiate a biloma from a chronic subcapsular hematoma or abscess.*

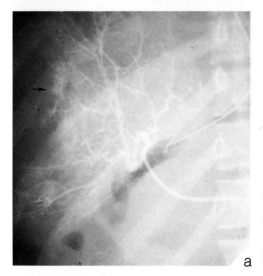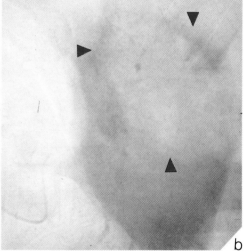

Fig. 9.8 Subcapsular hepatic hemorrhage.
a Ill-defined areas of contrast extravasation are seen along the lateral aspect of the right hepatic lobe. b The subtraction technique shows the extent of the hematoma (arrows). Note the compression of the normal parenchyma of the right lobe.

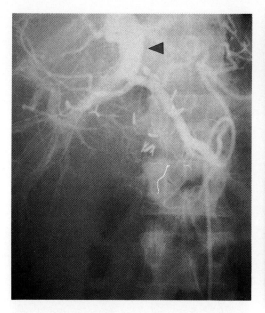

Fig. 9.9 Hepatic artery–portal vein arterio-venous fistula. *A selective hepatic arteri-ogram opacifies the portal vein (arrow), which should not normally occur. (The portal vein should be opacified only by contrast injection into the splenic or mesenteric vessels.) Hepatic artery–portal vein fistulas can cause portal hypertension.*

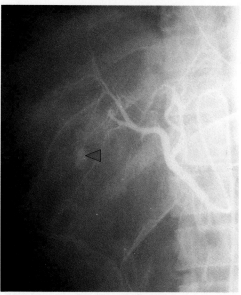

Fig. 9.10 Hepatic artery pseudoaneurysm. *A selective hepatic arteriogram in a patient with intraperitoneal bleeding shows extravasation of contrast material (arrow) from a branch of the right hepatic artery.*

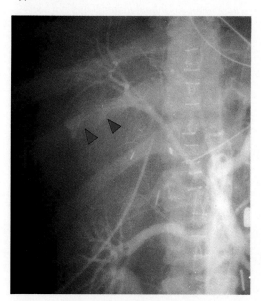

Fig. 9.11 Hepatic artery–bile duct fistula. *A celiac arteriogram in a patient with hemobilia shows extravasation of contrast material (arrows) into the biliary tree.*

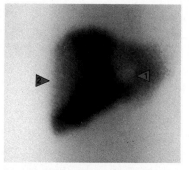

Fig. 9.12 Scintigraphic demon-stration of hepatic hematomas. *A TC^{99m} sulfur colloid scintiscan shows a photon-deficient area (arrow 1) representing an intra-parenchymal hematoma in the left lobe of the liver. Also note the con-cave lateral border of the right hep-atic lobe (arrow 2) due to a sub-capsular hematoma.*

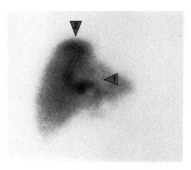

Fig. 9.13 Bile leak (lacerated bile duct). *TC⁹⁹ᵐ iminodiacetic acid (IDA) scintiscan demonstrates normal hepatic uptake and excretion of the radiopharmaceutical into the common bile duct (arrow 1). The "hot spot" over the dome of the liver (arrow 2) indicates a bile leak from a lacerated tributary of the right hepatic duct.*

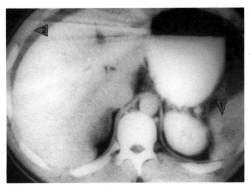

Fig. 9.14 Small intrasplenic hematoma. *Contrast-enhanced CT scan shows a low-attenuation area (arrow 1) in the center of the spleen. Note the hemoperitoneum (arrow 2) in the right subphrenic space.*

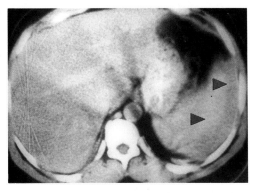

Fig. 9.15 Perisplenic hematoma. *A contrast-enhanced CT scan shows a low-attenuation area (arrows) surrounding the lateral aspect of the spleen. The border of the spleen is convex. If intravenous contrast material had not been administered, this hematoma might have gone unrecognized.*

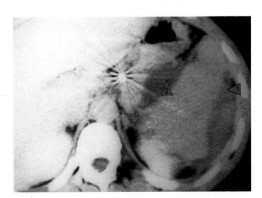

Fig. 9.16 Subcapsular splenic hematoma. *The lateral aspect of the spleen has a concave border caused by a subcapsular hematoma (arrow 1). Note the blood (arrow 2) in the lesser sac.*

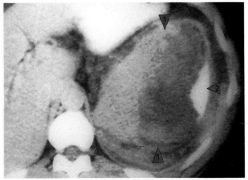

Fig. 9.17 Active subcapsular splenic hemorrhage. *Contrast-enhanced CT scan shows a low-attenuation subcapsular hematoma (arrows 1) displacing the splenic parenchyma medially. The lateral border of the spleen is concave. Lateral to the spleen is an area of very high attenuation (arrow 2) that represents active hemorrhage of contrast-enhanced blood.*

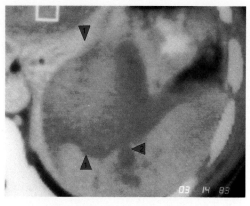

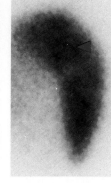

Fig. 9.19
Scintigraphic
demonstration of a
splenic hematoma.
*TC^{99m} sulfur colloid
scan shows a
photondeficient
area (arrow) at the
site of the splenic
hematoma.*

Fig. 9.18 Laceration of splenic hilus.
*Contrast-enhanced CT scan shows a large
hematoma in the lesser sac (arrows 1) and
several lacerations extending into the hilus of
the spleen (arrow 2).*

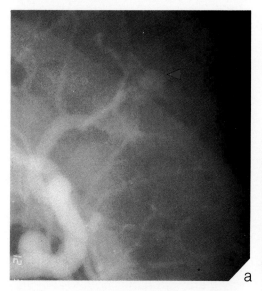

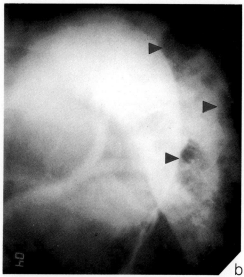

**Fig. 9.20 Angiographic evaluation of splenic
injury. *a* Celiac arteriogram shows active
bleeding from an upper lobar artery, manifested
by puddling of extravasated contrast material**
(arrow). ***b*** *In another patient, a selective
splenic arteriogram shows intrasplenic
hematomas (arrows) but no active bleeding.*

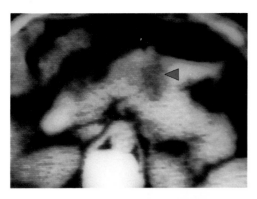

Fig. 9.21 Pancreatic hematoma. *Contrast-enhanced CT scan shows an area of decreased attenuation* (arrow) *in the body of the pancreas.*

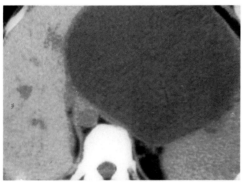

Fig. 9.22 Pancreatic pseudocyst. *Contrast-enhanced CT scan obtained 6 weeks after a blunt abdominal injury demonstrates a large water-density mass between the liver and spleen.*

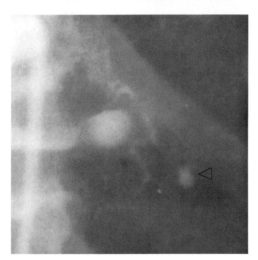

Fig. 9.23 Angiography of pancreatic trauma. *A celiac arteriogram in a patient who sustained a gunshot wound to the epigastrium shows extravasation* (arrow) *from a pancreatic branch of the splenic artery.*

INJURIES OF HOLLOW VISCERA

CT typically shows extravasation of the ingested contrast material in patients with rupture of the stomach (Fig. 9.24).

Injuries of the duodenum and jejunum are fre- quently difficult to appreciate on CT. The presence of retroperitoneal air and/or contrast material and a retroperitoneal or intramural hematoma strongly suggest a duodenal injury (Fig. 9.25), while free abdominal air and/or intraperitoneal leakage of

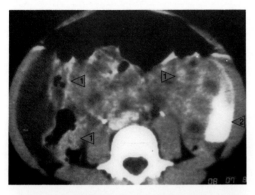

Fig. 9.24 Traumatic gastric rupture. *CT scan shows leakage of ingested contrast material into the peritoneal cavity. It can be seen between loops of bowel* (arrows 1) *and in the paracolic gutters* (arrow 2).

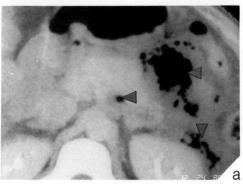

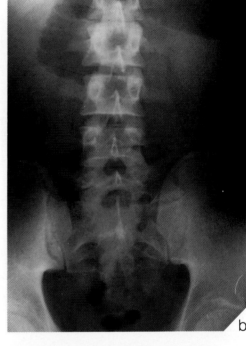

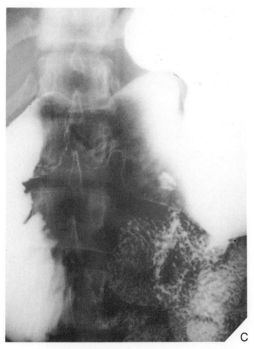

Fig. 9.25 Duodenal injuries. *a Contrast- enhanced CT scan in a patient with a traumatic perforation of the distal duodenum shows gas bubbles* (arrows) *in the retroperitoneum. b In another patient, a supine plain film shows dis- tension of the proximal duodenum with dimin- ished gas in the small bowel and colon. c A GI series shows partial obstruction of the trans- verse duodenum with a mass effect. This is a common location for traumatic duodenal hematomas.*

gastrointestinal contrast material is presumptive evidence of a jejunal or ileal perforation (Fig. 9.26). Colonic injuries are seldom detected by CT; a contrast enema is needed to diagnose them (Fig. 9.27). Penetrating injuries of the mesenteries typically lead to hematoma formation (Fig. 9.28). Injuries of the major mesenteric vessels may result in bowel ischemia (Fig. 9.29).

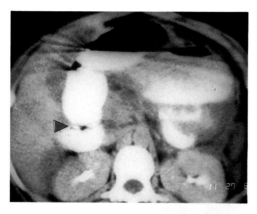

Fig. 9.26 Traumatic jejunal perforation. *CT scan shows a collection of contrast material* (arrow) *posterior to the stomach. Laparotomy revealed a perforation of the jejunum just beyond the ligament of Treitz.*

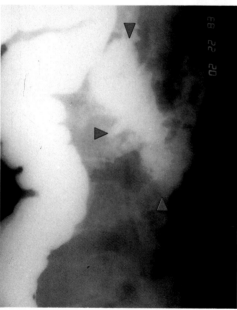

Fig. 9.27 Penetrating injury of the colon. *This patient with a stab wound of the left flank had a negative peritoneal lavage. A Gastrografin enema shows extravasation of contrast material* (arrows) *from the descending colon.*

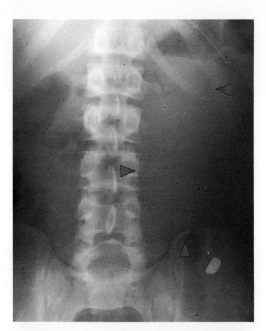

Fig. 9.28 Mesenteric hematoma. *A plain film of the abdomen shows a bullet in the left lower quadrant. The soft-tissue mass (arrows) to the left of the spine and cephalad to the bullet represents a large mesenteric hematoma.*

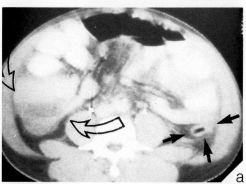

Fig. 9.29 Vascular injuries secondary to mesenteric trauma. *a CT shows marked distension of the proximal colon (open arrows) and collapse of the distal colon (closed arrows) secondary to traumatic occlusion of the inferior mesenteric artery with infarction of the left colon infarction. (This pattern might also be seen in colonic obstruction from other causes.) b Arteriogram in another patient shows a thrombus (arrow) in a branch of the inferior mesenteric artery.*

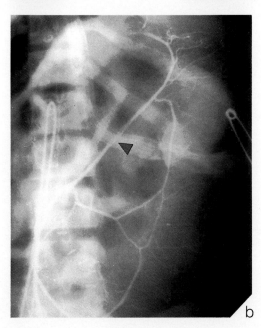

C H A P T E R   T E N

*I*njuries of the Retroperitoneum and Urinary Tract

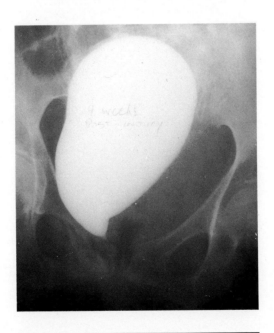

Imaging methods used to evaluate injuries of the kidneys, ureters, urinary tract, and urethra depend on the patient's hemodynamic status, the mechanism of injury, the presence and degree of hematuria, and whether or not other injuries are present. Available examinations include retrograde urethrography, intravenous urography, sonography, CT, and angiography.

PELVIC AND LOWER URINARY TRACT INJURIES

Retrograde urethrography should be performed in any stable male patient with a pelvic fracture who has signs or symptoms suggesting a urethral injury (e.g., inability to void, blood at the urethral meatus, and elevated, boggy prostate on rectal examination). If the patient is clinically stable, the urethrogram should be done prior to bladder catheterization to avoid further injury to the urethra. We obtain one or more oblique films of the urethra after injecting 10 ml of contrast material at the urethral meatus. Extravasation of contrast material at the base of the bladder indicates a posterior urethral injury; less severe injuries result in disruption of the supporting ligaments (Fig. 10.1).

Extravasation into the corpora of the penis indicates an anterior urethral injury (Fig. 10.2). Anterior and posterior urethral injuries may also result from penetrating wounds (Figs. 10.3–10.5).

Retrograde cystography is indicated in patients who present with hematuria after blunt lower abdominal or pelvic trauma or a gunshot wound to the pelvis. Bladder leaks may be intraperitoneal or extraperitoneal. To ensure that a small leak will not be overlooked, the bladder must be distended with at least 400 ml of contrast material; films are obtained both with the bladder filled and after draining the contrast material from the bladder via the catheter (Fig. 10.6). In intra-peritoneal leaks, contrast material can be identified in the cul-de-sac and the peritoneal cavity (Fig. 10.7). Extraperitoneal extravasation is localized around the bladder.

Extraperitoneal hematomas associated with pelvic fractures typically displace and elevate the bladder (Fig. 10.8). CT is very useful in the assessment of these injuries, which may be associated with extensive retroperitoneal bleeding (Figs. 10.9, 10.10).

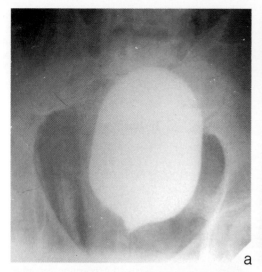

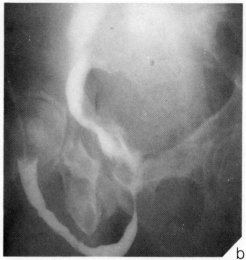

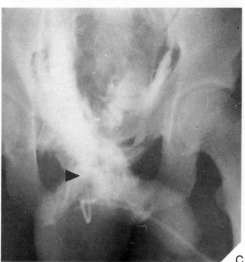

Fig. 10.1 Posterior urethral injuries. *a Type I injury: The cystogram shows elevation of the base of the bladder secondary to disruption of the prostatopubic ligaments. **b** Type II injury: In this type of posterior urethral injury, the laceration is above the urogenital diaphragm. The retrograde urethrogram shows extravasation of contrast material into the retroperitoneum. The fact that the extravasation is not seen below the membraneous urethra suggests that the urogenital diaphragm is intact. **c** Type III injury: In this type of injury the laceration involves the urogenital diaphragm. The retrograde urethrogram shows extravasation of contrast material into the pelvis and below the urogenital diaphragm (arrow indicates extravasation into the scrotum).*

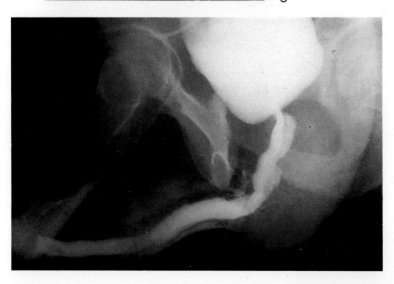

Fig. 10.2 Anterior urethral laceration. *A retrograde urethrogram shows extravasation of contrast material within the corpora of the penis. There is no extravasation into the perineum.*

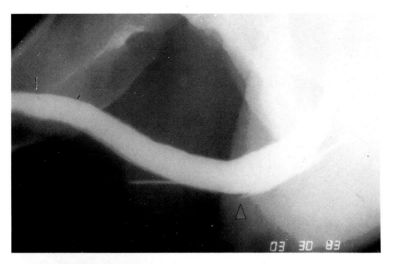

Fig. 10.3 Urethral foreign body. *This psychotic patient introduced a pin into his urethra and presented with hematuria. The retrograde urethrogram shows that the pin (arrow) has perforated the urethra.*

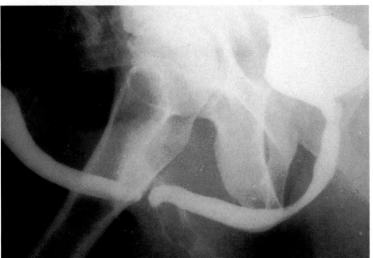

Fig. 10.4 Transection of anterior urethra. *This patient sustained a knife wound of the penis and was unable to void. A combined retrograde urethrogram and suprapubic cystogram (contrast material introduced via an indwelling suprapubic catheter) shows a gap in the penile urethra.*

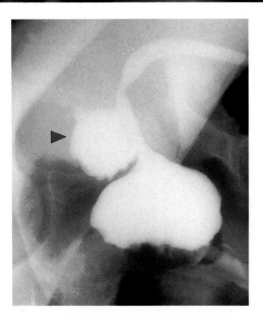

Fig. 10.5 Gunshot wound of the prostatic urethra. *A suprapubic cystourethrogram (contrast material introduced via an indwelling suprapubic catheter) in a patient with a gunshot wound shows extravasation from the prostatic urethra into a large cavity (arrow) in the prostatic fossa.*

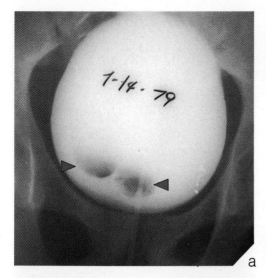

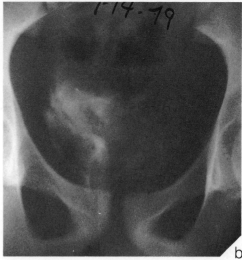

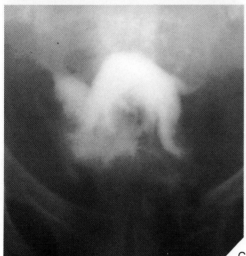

Fig. 10.6 Retroperitoneal bladder perforation. *a A film of the filled urinary bladder shows several filling defects* (arrows) *that represent blood clots. No extravasation is seen. **b** A repeat film obtained after emptying the bladder. Note the extravasated contrast material that had been masked by the distended, opacified bladder. **c** In another patient with a retroperitoneal bladder laceration, the postemptying film shows more extensive extravasation of contrast material.*

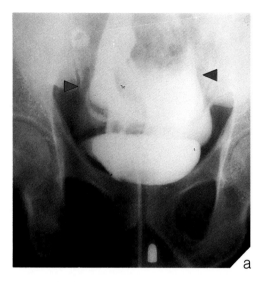

Fig. 10.7 Intraperitoneal bladder perforation.
*a A cystogram shows a collection of contrast
material* (arrows) *superior to the bladder, in the
pelvic cul-de-sac. b In another patient with an
intraperitoneal urine leak, a film of the
abdomen obtained after retrograde cystography shows extravasated contrast material outlining small bowel loops* (arrows 1). *Contrast
material is also seen in the left subphrenic
space* (arrow 2).

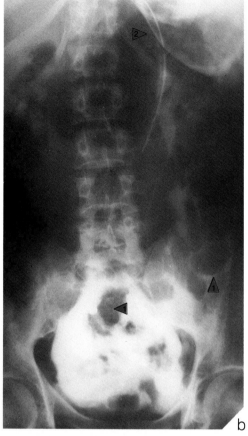

Fig. 10.8 Perivesical hematoma. *Retrograde
cystogram in a patient with a pelvic fracture.
The bladder is displaced to the right and
elevated by a retroperitoneal hematoma.*

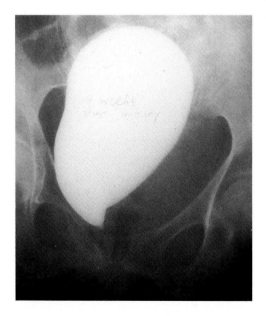

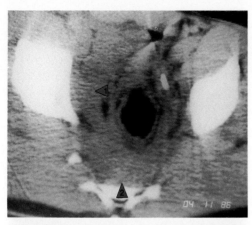

Fig. 10.9 Pelvic retroperitoneal hematomas.
*CT in a patient with a pelvic fractures shows a
hematoma (arrow 1)* medial to the right acetabulum, displacing the rectum to the left, which is
presumably due to a laceration of the obturator
artery. In addition, the rectum is displaced
anteriorly by a presacral hematoma (arrow 2),
presumably caused by bleeding from the
lateral sacral arteries.

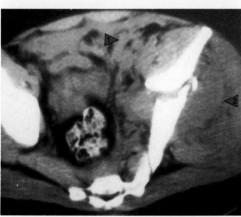

**Fig. 10.10 Pelvic retroperitoneal
hematomas.** *In this patient, CT shows
hematomas (arrows 1 and 2)* on each side of
the fractured iliac wing. Iliacus hematomas
(arrow 1) and gluteal hematomas *(arrow 2)*
usually result from lacerations of the superior
gluteal artery.

UPPER URINARY TRACT AND RETROPERITONEAL INJURIES

Intravenous urography has traditionally been the initial radiologic examination in patients with suspected injuries of the retroperitoneum and upper urinary tract; however, intravenous urography provides limited information and the findings are often nonspecific (Figs. 10.11, 10.12). CT—which assesses renal perfusion, localizes renal and retroperitoneal hematomas, detects urine leakage, and identifies associated intraperitoneal and retroperitoneal injuries—is much more informative. At our institution, the evaluation of a patient with a suspected retroperitoneal hemorrhage and/or upper tract injury generally begins with contrast-enhanced CT (Figs. 10.13–10.24). Intravenous urography is reserved for unstable patients with blunt injuries and patients with penetrating wounds (Fig. 10.25).

Arteriography is indicated in patients with absent perfusion on IVU (Fig. 10.26) or active bleeding (Fig. 10.27). A traumatic arteriovenous fistula is an occasional late sequela of a renal injury (Fig. 10.28).

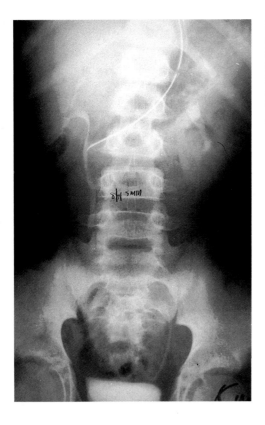

Fig. 10.11 Renal fracture. *This patient presented with hematuria following blunt trauma to the left flank. Intravenous urography shows good perfusion, and excretion on the left; neither renal outline is seen well. Angiography showed complete transection of the kidney with active bleeding. Nephrectomy was ultimately required.*

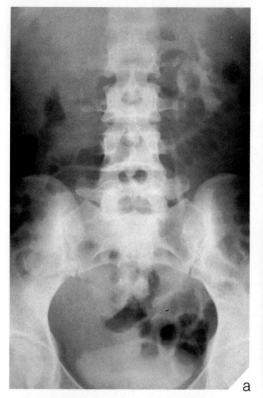

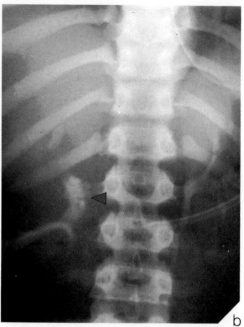

Fig. 10.12 Renal fracture. *This patient sustained blunt trauma to the right flank.* ***a*** *An early film from an IVU shows no excretion from the right kidney. This finding could be due to a contusion, renal vascular injury, renal fracture, an absent or diseased kidney, or a perinephric or subcapsular hematoma.* ***b*** *A later film shows extravasation of contrast material (arrow) from the right renal pelvis. There is a nephrogram in the upper half of the kidney and the upper pole calyces are opacified; there is no evidence of excretion in the devitalized lower half of the kidney.*

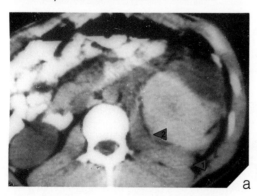

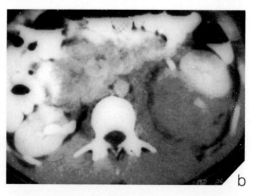

Fig. 10.13 Perinephric hematoma. ***a*** *An unenhanced CT scan shows a high-attenuation hematoma (arrow 1) posterior to the kidney. The psoas muscle (arrow 2) is well delineated. The hematoma, which is contained by the Gerota's fascia, is more dense than the kidney because no intravenous contrast material has been given.* ***b*** *On the contrast-enhanced CT scan, the hematoma is less dense than the kidney. The density of the hematoma has not changed but the density of the renal parenchyma has increased.*

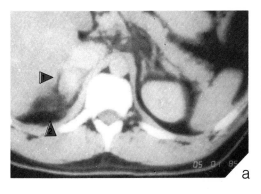 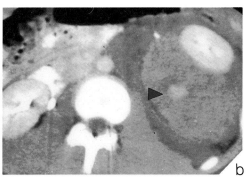

Fig. 10.14 Perinephric hematoma. *a* *Contrast-enhanced CT scan shows enlargement of the right adrenal gland* (arrow 1) *and increased density (due to hemorrhage) of the perinephric fat* (arrow 2) *lateral to the adrenal gland. In this patient, the perinephric hematoma is secondary to an adrenal injury.* ***b*** *Contrast-enhanced CT in* another patient demonstrates a large hematoma displacing the left kidney anteriorly. The small high-attenuation area (arrow) in the center of the hematoma represents an active arterial hemorrhage. The CT findings indicate a perinephric hematoma with active arterial bleeding (see Fig. 10.27).

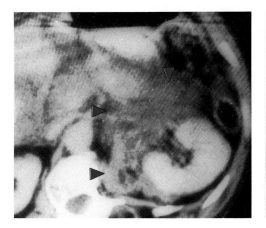 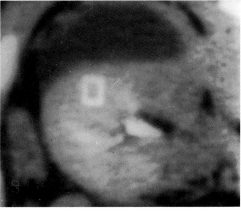

Fig. 10.15 Central perinephric hematoma. *Contrast-enhanced CT scan shows a hematoma medial to the left kidney (arrows). The location of the hematoma suggests a vascular injury. This patient had avulsed tributaries of the renal vein.*

Fig. 10.16 Subcapsular hematoma. *Contrast-enhanced CT shows a hematoma posterior to the kidney. Because of its intracapsular location, the hematoma causes a concavity in the margin of the kidney, similar to that seen in subcapsular hematomas of the liver and spleen.*

Fig. 10.17 Posterior pararenal hematoma. *On this contrast-enhanced CT scan, the right psoas muscle (arrow) is enlarged and ill-defined compared to the left psoas. This hematoma was caused by a laceration of a lumbar artery.*

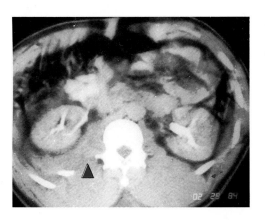

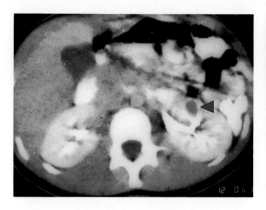

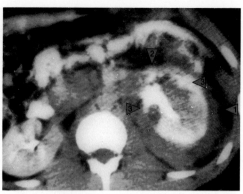

Fig. 10.18 Intrarenal hematoma. *Contrast-enhanced CT shows a low-attenuation area (arrow) surrounded by enhanced renal parenchyma. There is no urinary leakage or extrarenal hemorrhage. This appearance is compatible with a renal hematoma, tumor, or cyst. A follow-up CT would help to establish the correct diagnosis.*

Fig. 10.19 Renal fracture. *Contrast-enhanced CT shows a perinephric hematoma (arrow 1), urine extravasation (arrow 2), increased enhancement of the left kidney compared to the right (due to stasis), and low-attenuation areas (arrows 3) within the renal parenchyma. These findings indicate a fracture of the left kidney.*

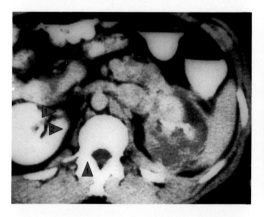

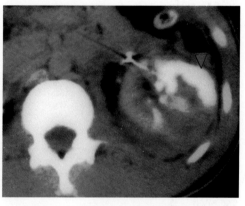

Fig. 10.20 Renal fracture with urinoma formation. *Contrast-enhanced CT shows a fluid collection (arrows 1) surrounding the upper pole of the right kidney. Note that contrast material is actively leaking into the urinoma (arrow 2).*

Fig. 10.21 Perinephric urine leak. *Following operative repair of a gunshot wound of the left kidney, CT shows leakage of contrast material (arrow) anterior to the kidney, into the perinephric space.*

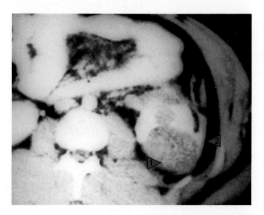

Fig. 10.22 Renal transection with intraperitoneal urinary leak. *Contrast-enhanced CT shows the absence of enhancement in the lower pole of the left kidney (arrow 1). Contrast-enhanced urine (arrow 2) is seen anterior to the devascularized segment, extending into the paracolic gutter.*

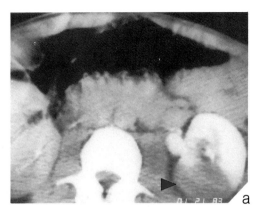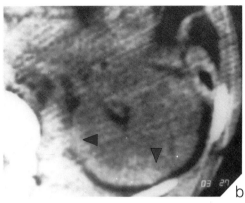

Fig. 10.23 Renal artery occlusion. *a Contrast-enhanced CT shows nonenhancement of the posterior portion of the left kidney (arrow) due to occlusion of a segmental artery. **b** In a patient with complete occlusion of the left renal artery, contrast-enhanced CT shows the absence of enhancement and the absence of excretion in the affected kidney. Note the cortical enhancement (arrows), which represents cortical perfusion by capsular collaterals.*

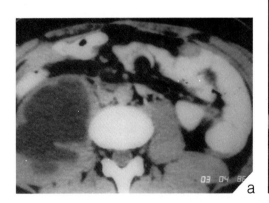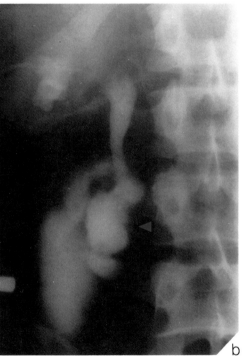

Fig. 10.24 Ureteral Injury. *a Unenhanced CT following surgical repair of a lacerated ureter shows a large urine collection in the right psoas region. **b** An antegrade nephrostomy study demonstrates leakage of urine (arrow) at the site of the repair. Ureteral injuries are rare. Most are iatrogenic (e.g., intraoperative trauma, and stone–basket manipulation). Ureteral injuries are occasionally caused by penetrating injuries but are rarely seen after blunt trauma.*

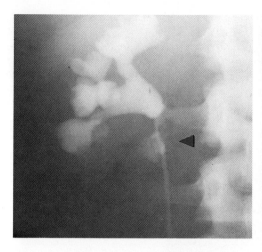

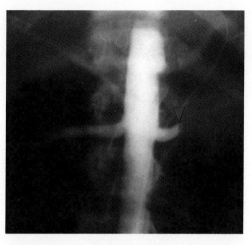

Fig. 10.25 Ureteral injury. *IVU in a patient with a gunshot wound of the abdomen demonstrates leakage of urine from the proximal ureter (arrow) and dilatation of the renal collecting system.*

Fig. 10.26 Renal artery occlusion. *Aortogram demonstrates an abrupt cutoff of the proximal left renal artery (arrow).*

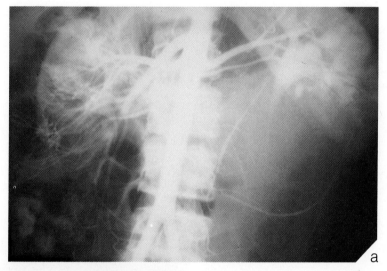

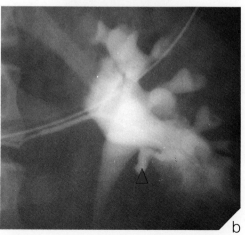

Fig. 10.27 Active renal bleeding into the retroperitoneum. *a An aortogram shows a large mass effect. The aorta is displaced to the right and the left kidney is displaced upward and laterally. b A selective left renal arteriogram shows active arterial bleeding (arrow) from a lacerated accessory renal artery (see also Fig. 10.14b).*

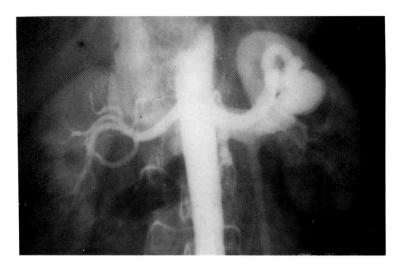

Fig. 10.28 Renal arteriovenous fistula. *This patient had a kidney injury 30 years before. An aortogram shows enlargement of the left renal artery, a varix in the upper pole of the left kidney, and early opacification of the left renal vein and inferior vena cava. There is reflux into the left gonadal vein.*

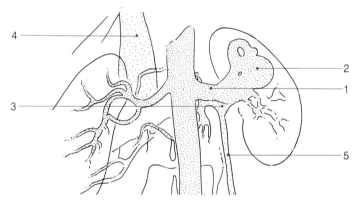

1 Enlarged left renal artery
2 Varix in upper pole of left kidney
3 Left renal vein

4 Inferior vena cava
5 Left gonadal vein

CHAPTER ELEVEN

Vascular Trauma

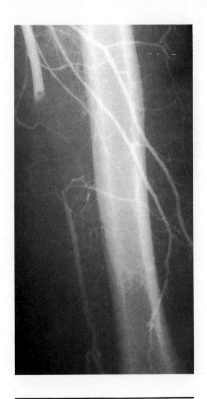

Arteriography plays an important role in the management of vascular trauma. It can exclude vascular injury and avoid unnecessary surgical exploration (Figs. 11.1, 11.2). Accurate characterization and localization of vascular injuries facilitates treatment planning. Moreover, bleeding can occasionally be controlled using percutaneous transcatheter embolization techniques.

The main indications for arteriography are (1) a large or expanding hematoma; (2) a pulse deficit (Figs. 11.2–11.5); and (3) a penetrating wound in proximity to a major vessel (Figs. 11.6–11.10). Certain injuries may indicate the need for emergency arteriography. Aortography is commonly done to exclude aortic rupture in patients who have sustained decelerating thoracic trauma (Fig. 11.11), while knee dislocation is an indication for popliteal arteriography. Loss of pulses after a supracondylar fracture of the humerus is a frequent indication for emergency brachial arteriography, especially in children (see Figs. 11.1, 11.2).

Multiple views and serial films are essential for the accurate assessment of a vascular injury. If possible, the examination should be done by a radiologist under fluoroscopic guidance in a well-equipped special procedure suite. Single-view ("one-shot") emergency-room arteriography should be avoided.

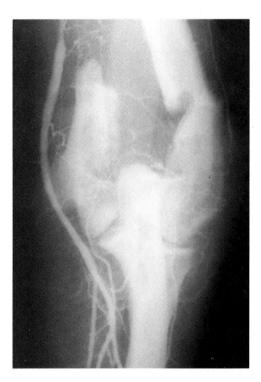

Fig. 11.1 Mass effect. *The brachial artery is displaced around a displaced bone fragment in this patient with a comminuted intercondylar fracture of the humerus. No vascular injury is seen. Similar vascular displacement might also be caused by a hematoma.*

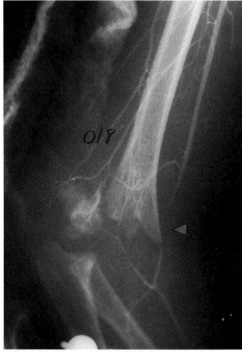

Fig. 11.2 Arterial spasm. *In this child with a supracondylar fracture of the humerus, the brachial artery is patent but markedly narrowed at the fracture site (arrow). Spasm is most commonly seen in the upper extremity and in children, but it may occur in any injured artery and at any age. It is difficult to exclude true arterial injury when marked spasm is present.*

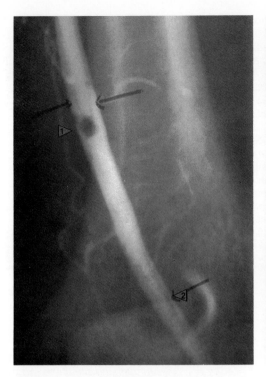

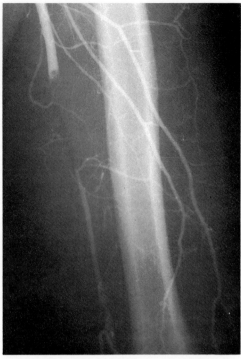

Fig. 11.3 Mural thrombus and intimal dissection. *The radiolucent filling defect (arrow 1) within the arterial lumen seen on this brachial arteriogram represents a "platelet" plug adherent to the site of intimal injury. The linear filling defects (arrow 2) represent dissected intima.*

Fig. 11.4 Arterial thrombosis. *In this patient with a gunshot wound of the thigh, the brachial artery is thrombosed and is opacified distal to the point of obstruction by collaterals. It cannot be determined from this arteriogram whether the underlying vascular injury is a transection, laceration, or intimal injury.*

Fig. 11.5 Bullet embolism. *In this patient with a gunshot wound of the chest, a chest film failed to demonstrate the bullet. Distal pulses were absent in the right leg. A femoral arteriogram shows the bullet (arrow) occluding the superficial femoral artery in the midthigh. After entering the chest, the bullet had penetrated the left ventricle and embolized to the superficial femoral artery.*

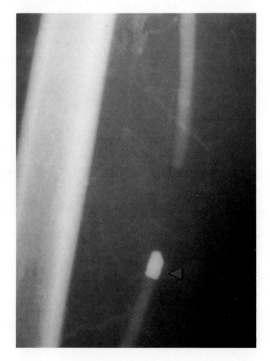

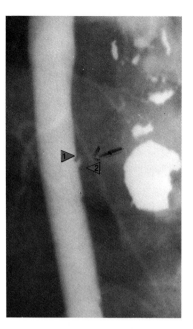

Fig. 11.6 Gunshot wound of the internal carotid artery. *In this patient with a penetrating neck wound, a carotid arteriogram shows an intimal flap (arrow 1) and a localized bulge of contrast material (arrow 2) in the vessel wall. Irregularities, narrowing, outpockets of the contrast column, and linear filling defects are seen with incomplete mural injuries. Such lesions are usually associated with high-velocity gunshot wounds (which may not have penetrated the vessel) and blunt stretch injuries. (see also Fig. 11.11).*

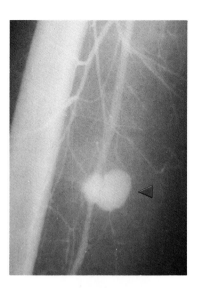

Fig. 11.7 Incomplete arterial laceration. *In this patient with a gunshot wound of the thigh, a femoral arteriogram shows extravasation of contrast material (arrow). Because there is continuity of flow through the site of the extravasation, an incomplete laceration of the vessel can be diagnosed.*

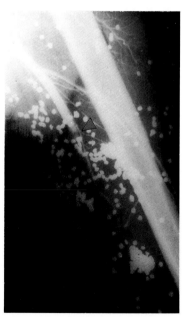

Fig. 11.8 Shotgun wound. *A femoral arteriogram shows thrombosis of the superficial femoral artery (arrow) in this patient with a shotgun wound. Shotgun wounds are widespread and the vessel may be injured at multiple sites. Because it is extremely difficult to plan an operative approach to the vessel without arteriography, this study should be done in all stable patients who sustain shotgun wounds of an extremity.*

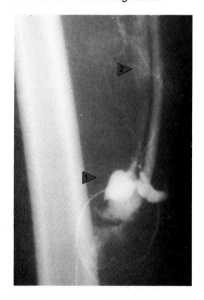

Fig. 11.9 Acute arteriovenous fistula. *An early film from a femoral arteriogram in a patient with a gunshot wound of the thigh shows extravasation (arrow 1) from the superficial femoral artery and simultaneous filling of the femoral vein (arrow 2), which runs parallel to the artery.*

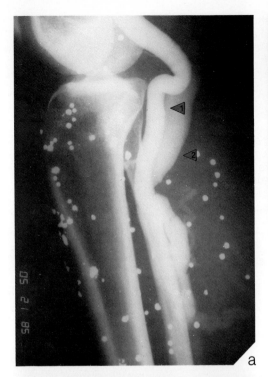

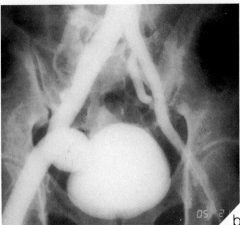

Fig. 11.10 Chronic arteriovenous fistula. *a,*
b A femoral arteriogram in a patient who sus-
tained a shotgun wound of the right calf several
months before shows a fistula between the
popliteal artery (arrow 1) and the popliteal vein
(arrow 2). All of the vessels of the right lower
extremity are dilated and tortuous, both at the
site of the fistula (a) and more proximally (b).

Fig. 11.11 Aortic arch intimal injury. *This*
patient, who sustained blunt thoracic trauma,
had a fracture of the first rib. An aortic arch
injection shows an intimal injury associated
with bulging of the contrast column (arrow)
(see also Fig. 11.6).

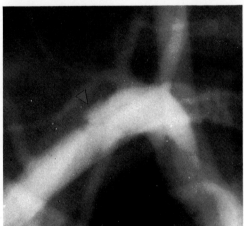

INDEX